Pocket Book of Food Facts

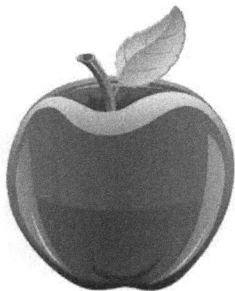

Fruits

And

Vegetables

Evelyne Mindes MD

Pocket Book of Food Facts

FRUITS AND VEGETABLES
Legumes, Nuts and Seeds

Evelyne Mindes MD

Internal Medicine

Justin Press Publishing

An entity of

Keto Enterprises West Inc.
P.O. Box 24110
Los Angeles Calif. 90024

Justin Press Publishing is an entity under the fictitious name of Keto Enterprises West Inc. of Los Angeles California. P.O. BOX 24110, Los Angeles California 90024

Printed in the USA

ISBN: 10: 09978352-1-4
ISBN: 13: 978-0-9978352-1-2

Evelyne Mindes MD received an Associate of Arts and a Bachelor's Degree from UCLA, a Master's Degree from George Williams College of Chicago Illinois, and the degree of Doctor of Medicine from UCLA. As a practicing Internist, she had the opportunity to expand her interest in diet and nutrition.

HOW TO USE THIS BOOK

I began developing this booklet many years ago. Since then research and nutritional knowledge has progressed. The nomenclature, and even the specifics have changed. Originally I used the RDA meaning Recommended Daily Allowance as a basis for comparison. Today, the research and literature speak more about the *Dietary Reference Intake. (DRI),* rather than the RDA. The numbers provided herein come from many different sources and not all sources agree on the exact same number. Anyone needing or wanting specific information about any element should go to one of the resources listed at the back of this booklet. I specifically recommend the *NATIONAL ACADEMY OF SCIENCE* and the USDA References. The material is detailed and voluminous.

The reader/user of the material on these pages, **SHOULD NOT RELY ON ANY SPECIFIC VALUE SHOWN HEREIN.** The intent of this booklet is to give the reader an *idea* of the nutrient value of a specific fruit, seed, or vegetable. These numbers are a *guide* for making choice, and should **NOT** be used as an absolute basis for making critical nutritional decisions. Each individual as well as each item and or circumstance will be different.

Eat What You Want……….YEAH………. it's the calories

Hear we go again…another Eating Guide… and to top it off, I claim that you really can "Eat what you want" and still lose weight. After all, that is what MILLIONS of normal weight people do every day. They are not fixated daily on food. So-o-o- what is the catch? The catch is that they do not eat more than _their_ body uses. So no matter what ANY diet plan or advice says. There has to be a balance and it is individual.. But then, that is the **GOOD NEWS.** It means that you really can eat almost anything _you_ want.

Yes, theoretically you could have expensive chocolates, day after day. You could eat Turkey and dressing and cream cheese pies for dessert if you wanted to….that is as long as **you** did not exceed the amount of food _your_ body used up. **HOWEVER,** I did not say that you might not, _rot out your teeth or die of malnutrition_ !!! …….but that's the **BAD NEWS .**

But…. back to basics, and my original tenet. IT'S THE CALORIES! That makes it the GOOD NEWS because some times, we have a choice. The BAD NEWS is that many of us are conditioned by genes, habits, family eating patterns, "food additions" etc, so that to some extent eating becomes difficult

This booklet repeats the information that you can find in any book on foods or nutrition. The goal here is of choice. To maintain a healthy weight you must balance intake. The first key is KNOWLEDGE. This book attempts to aid in that respect

The second key is readiness. This is partially a head-trip; perhaps, the most difficult For many, it is going to require a total change in attitude and comfort regarding food. The "average " normal" weight person does not "live to eat". …instead….. they " eat to live" and consume only what is needed to sustain life. An "Eat What You Want" diet may leave you nutritionally unbalanced and require high quality multiple vitamin supplements. Fruits, vegetables and seeds are often high in fiber, and water but low in fat and total calories. For example, an entire head of iceberg lettuce is, though low in total nutrients, probably only 70 kilocalories. Whereas, one McDonald's "Big Mac"® is said to contain approximately 560 calories![1] Use this as a guide to help you attain your goal of a balanced and nutritional food intake.

---

[1] McDonald's Nutrition Facts: McDonald Nutrition Information Center Booklet published by the McDonald Corporation 1997

CAL: 31

Type: Fruit

Size: 1 cup

Description: This fruit comes from a small bushy tree even though it can grow up to 15 feet tall. It has been a native of the West Indies, Mexico, Central and South America. This fruit has also been known as the Puerto Rican, West Indian or Barbados Cherry. Tart in taste, this small berry is similar in appearance to a cherry. It is red in color when ripe and has a soft flesh. It has been considered a good source of vitamin C, maintaining a high level of this even when prepared as a jelly.

NUTRIENTS:

Carbohydrates				7.54	gms
Proteins				0.39	gms
Fats				0.29	mg
	Cholesterol			0	mg
	Saturated				
Water				90	%
Fiber				0.39	gms
Minerals					
	Calcium			12	mg
	Iron			0.20	mg
	Magnesium			18	mg
Vitamins					
	A			751	I.U
	B1			0.02	mg
	B2			0.06	mg
	Niacin			0.39	mg
	B6				
	B12				mcg
	C			1,644	mg
	D				I.U
	E				I.U
	Folic acid				mcg
	K				mcg
Electrolytes					
	Sodium			7	mg
	Potassium			143	mg

13

ALFALFA SPROUTS   CAL 10

Type ; Vegetable - seed

Size: 1 cup raw

Description: This seed comes from a perennial plant and under proper conditions the plant will live from three to six or more years. The seeds are kidney shaped and develop inside small twisted or cured pods. The plant has been used for any years as a crop for animals. Today the sprouts are popular in cooked dishes and in salads

NUTRIENTS:

Carbohydrates				1	gms
Proteins				1	gms
Fats				tr	mg
	Cholesterol			0	mg
	Saturated			tr	
Water				91	%
Fiber					gms
Minerals					
	Calcium			11	mg
	Iron			0.3	mg
	Magnesium				mg
Vitamins					
	A			50	I.U
	B1			0.03	mg
	B2			0.04	mg
	Niacin			0.2	mg
	B6				
	B12				mcg
	C			3	mg
	D				I.U
	E				I.U
	Folic acid				mcg
	K				mcg
Electrolytes					
	Sodium			2	mg
	Potassium			26	mg

CAL : 135

Type: Seed

Size: 1 oz whole

Description: This is the seed or fruit of the Almond tree which grows widely: California, Australia, Southern Europe and Asia are common locations. The tree looks very similar to the Peach tree and the seed or kernel is also similar in appearance and taste. They are either bitter or sweet by taste and thin or hard in shell quality. The variety can be pealed with just the finger. Years ago, they were named by the country of origin but it is not known if that custom still persists today. One type, the Jordan Almond is usually larger and has a more delicate flavor than others. Almonds are eaten fresh, made into meal for cooking purposes, and the oil is extracted for many uses.

NUTRIENTS:

Carbohydrates				6	gms
Proteins				6	gms
Fats				15	mg
	Cholesterol			0	mg
	Saturated			1.4	gms
Water				4	%
Fiber					gms
Minerals					
	Calcium			75	mg
	Iron			1.0	mg
	Magnesium				mg
Vitamins					
	A			0	I.U
	B1			0.06	mg
	B2			0.33	mg
	Niacin			1.0	mg
	B6				
	B12				mcg
	C			tr	mg
	D				I.U
	E				I.U
	Folic acid				mcg
	K				mcg
Electrolytes					
	Sodium			3	mg
	Potassium			208	mg

Type: Fruit

Size: medium

Description: Many varieties, Delicious, Golden Delicious, Granny, Gravenstein, Fuji, Jonathan , McIntosh, Pippins, Rome etc. Most are commonly eaten raw entirely. Pippins are quite tart and generally used in cooking. The apple belongs to the rose family as are pears, cherries, peaches, and plums. There is a variety of wild apple called the crab apple. It is a hard, small sour fruit which when eaten, is most commonly made into jams or jellies. The apple supplies pectin which is good for the digestion. .

NUTRIENTS:

Carbohydrates				21	gms
Proteins				tr	gms
Fats				tr	mg
	Cholesterol			0	mg
	Saturated			0.1	
Water				84	%
Fiber				1.06	gms
Minerals					
	Calcium			10	mg
	Iron			0.2	mg
	Magnesium			6	mg
Vitamins					
	A			70	I.U
	B1			0.02	mg
	B2			0.02	mg
	Niacin			0.01	mg
	B6			.06	mg
	B12			0	mcg
	C			8	mg
	D				I.U
	E				I.U
	Folic acid			3.9	mcg
	K				mcg
Electrolytes					
	Sodium			tr	mg
	Potassium			159	mg

CAL : 50   **APRICOTS**

Type: Fruit

Size: Three small

Description: Smaller in size and purer in yellow color. These fruits resemble peaches. They do not hold up well as a raw fruit and therefore many are dried or canned. The dry sulfured form is richer in Vitamin A than the other forms and is considered a good source of this vitamin.

NUTRIENTS:

Carbohydrates				12	gms
Proteins				1	gms
Fats				tr	mg
	Cholesterol			0	mg
	Saturated			tr	
Water				86	%
Fiber				.64	gms
Minerals					
	Calcium			15	mg
	Iron			0.6	mg
	Magnesium			8	mg
Vitamins					
	A			2,770	I.U
	B1			0.03	mg
	B2			0.04	mg
	Niacin			0.6	mg
	B6			0.06	
	B12				mcg
	C			11	mg
	D				I.U
	E			9.1	I.U
	Folic acid				mcg
	K				mcg
Electrolytes					
	Sodium			1	mg
	Potassium			314	mEq

ARTICHOLES   CAL:35

Type: Vegetable

Size: 1 whole cooked ....French

Description: The plant is a perennial which produces new buds yearly, usually in the summer. The part that is commonly eaten is harvested beginning in the fall. The globe artichoke is a member of the thistle family. And has been known since the early 18th century. The fleshy part of the petal is the part eaten but the hearts are also favorites. The major portion of the leaf is quite fibrous and is discarded. The edible part is usually dipped in either butter or a sauce.

NUTRIENTS:

Carbohydrates				12	gms
Proteins				3	gms
Fats				tr	mg
	Cholesterol			0	mg
	Saturated			tr	
Water				87	%
Fiber				1.5	gms
Minerals					
	Calcium			47	mg
	Iron			1.6	mg
	Magnesium			76	mg
Vitamins					
	A			170	I.U
	B1			0.07	mg
	B2			0.6	mg
	Niacin			1.2	mg
	B6			.13	
	B12			0	mcg
	C			11,9	mg
	D				I.U
	E				I.U
	Folic acid			6.1	mcg
	K				mcg
Electrolytes					
	Sodium			79	mg
	Potassium			316	mg

ARUGULA

Type: Vegetable

Size: ½ cup

Description: These leaves have become a common ingredient in salads. For some the taste is slightly bitter.

NUTRIENTS:

Carbohydrates				0.36	gms
Proteins				0.26	gms
Fats				0.07	mg
	Cholesterol			0	mg
	Saturated			0	
Water				91	%
Fiber				0	gms
Minerals					
	Calcium			16	mg
	Iron				mg
	Magnesium			5	mg
Vitamins					
	A			237	I.U
	B1			0.004	mg
	B2			0.009	mg
	Niacin			0.030	mg
	B6			0.007	
	B12			0	mcg
	C			0	mg
	D				I.U
	E				I.U
	Folic acid			10	mcg
	K				mcg
Electrolytes					
	Sodium			3	mg
	Potassium			37	mg

19

ASPARAGUS

Type: Vegetable

Size: 1 cup

Description: There are two types of this Lily of the Valley family member: green and white. The white has a thicker stem and usually only the tip is eaten whereas all of the stem of the green is eaten.. A clue to the freshness of the green variety is that its stalk is perfectly straight and the scales at the tips are closely pressed and taper to a point. As the stalks age the scales dry and stand out from each other. The lower part of the stalk of the white variety becomes dry and pithy as it gets older.

NUTRIENTS:

Carbohydrates				3	gms
Proteins				2	gms
Fats				tr	mg
	Cholesterol			0	mg
	Saturated			tr	
Water				92	%
Fiber				0.50	gms
Minerals					
	Calcium			14	mg
	Iron			0.4	mg
	Magnesium			6	mg
Vitamins					
	A			2	I.U
	B1			0.06	mg
	B2			0.07	mg
	Niacin			0.6	mg
	B6			0.7	
	B12			0	mcg
	C			16	mg
	D				I.U
	E				I.U
	Folic acid			88	mcg
	K			48	mcg
Electrolytes					
	Sodium			2	mg
	Potassium			186	mg

Type: Fruit

Size: 1 medium (approximately ½ LB)

Description: though technically a fruit because it is not sweet, many consider it a vegetable. There are several varieties. It is commonly grown in California, Florida, and Mexico. It is usually eaten raw, alone or in salads. Often it is made into a sauce called Guacemole. Some times it is called by other names such as Alligator Pear, and Calvado. It comes in one of three shapes, pear, oval or round.

NUTRIENTS:

Carbohydrates				12	gms
Proteins				4	gms
Fats				30	mg
	Cholesterol			0	mg
	Saturated			4.5	
Water				73	%
Fiber				4.24	gms
Minerals					
	Calcium			19	mg
	Iron			2.0	mg
	Magnesium			79	mg
Vitamins					
	A			1,060	I.U
	B1			0.19	mg
	B2			0.21	mg
	Niacin			3.3	mg
	B6			0.56	
	B12			0	mcg
	C			14	mg
	D				I.U
	E				I.U
	Folic acid			124.4	mcg
	K				mcg
Electrolytes					
	Sodium				mg
	Potassium				mg

BAMBOO SHOOTS   CAL: 35

Type: Vegetable

Size: 1 cup canned, dried

Description: The Bamboo tree produces an underground root, that when out of the ground reveals young shoots which are tightly surrounded. It is the inner white shoots, which are cooked when the outer covering is removed. These shoots are prepared in several ways, boiled in salted water, fried etc. For years they have been commonly found in Japanese and Chinese cooking.

NUTRIENTS:

Carbohydrates				4	gms
Proteins				2	gms
Fats				1	mg
	Cholesterol			0	mg
	Saturated			0.1	
Water				94	%
Fiber					gms
Minerals					
	Calcium			10	mg
	Iron			0.4	mg
	Magnesium				mg
Vitamins					
	A			10	I.U
	B1			0.03	mg
	B2			0.03	mg
	Niacin			0.2	mg
	B6				
	B12				mcg
	C			1	mg
	D				I.U
	E				I.U
	Folic acid				mcg
	K				mcg
Electrolytes					
	Sodium			9	mg
	Potassium			105	mg

Type: Fruit

Size: 1 (approximately ¼ lb)

Description: Grow on a stalk usually spoken of as a "hand". The usual variety eaten raw, is yellow in color though picked green. Many think it is at its best flavor and sweetness when flecked with brown. There is a variety called "plaintain" which is not as sweet. It is rarely eaten raw and when cooked resembles a potato in texture.

NUTRIENTS:

Carbohydrates				27	gms
Proteins				1	gms
Fats				1	mg
	Cholesterol			0	mg
	Saturated			0.2	
Water				74	%
Fiber				.57	gms
Minerals					
	Calcium			7	mg
	Iron			0.4	mg
	Magnesium			33	mg
Vitamins					
	A			90	I.U
	B1			0.05	mg
	B2			11	mg
	Niacin			0.6	mg
	B6			0.66	
	B12			0	mcg
	C			10	mg
	D				I.U
	E				I.U
	Folic acid			21.8	mcg
	K				mcg
Electrolytes					
	Sodium			1	mg
	Potassium			451	mg

BEANS, BLACK   **CAL:225**

Type: Legume

Size: 1 cup cooked

Description: Beans in general, are higher in protein than most other vegetables. They are frequently described by their color. A FEW are listed herein separately due to the few variations in their nutritive values

NUTRIENTS:

Carbohydrates				41	gms
Proteins				15	gms
Fats				1	mg
	Cholesterol			0	mg
	Saturated			0.1	
Water				66	%
Fiber					gms
Minerals					
	Calcium			47	mg
	Iron			2.9	mg
	Magnesium				mg
Vitamins					
	A			tr	I.U
	B1			0.43	mg
	B2			0.05	mg
	Niacin			0.9	mg
	B6				
	B12				mcg
	C			0	mg
	D				I.U
	E				I.U
	Folic acid				mcg
	K				mcg
Electrolytes					
	Sodium			1	mg
	Potassium			608	mg

24

CAL: 210   **BEANS, GREAT NORTHERN**

Type: Legume

Size: 1 cup cooked

Description: Beans in general are higher in protein than other vegetables. The Great Northern Bean is usually white in color.

Carbohydrates				38	gms
Proteins				14	gms
Fats				1	mg
	Cholesterol			0	mg
	Saturated			0.1	
Water				69	%
Fiber					gms
Minerals					
	Calcium			90	mg
	Iron			4.9	mg
	Magnesium				mg
Vitamins					
	A			0	I.U
	B1			0.25	mg
	B2			0.13	mg
	Niacin			1.3	mg
	B6				
	B12				mcg
	C			0	mg
	D				I.U
	E				I.U
	Folic acid				mcg
	K				mcg
Electrolytes					
	Sodium			13	mg
	Potassium			749	mg

25

Type: Legume

Size: 1 cup cooked

Description: Beans in general are higher in protein than other vegetables. They vary in color and amount of nutrients according to variety.

NUTRIENTS:

Carbohydrates				49	gms
Proteins				16	gms
Fats				1	mg
	Cholesterol			0	mg
	Saturated			0.2	
Water				64	%
Fiber					gms
Minerals					
	Calcium			55	mg
	Iron			5.9	mg
	Magnesium				mg
Vitamins					
	A			tr	I.U
	B1			0.25	mg
	B2			0.11	mg
	Niacin			1.3	mg
	B6				
	B12				mcg
	C			0	mg
	D				I.U
	E				I.U
	Folic acid				mcg
	K				mcg
Electrolytes					
	Sodium			4	mg
	Potassium			1,163	mg

Type: Legume

Size: 1 cup cooked

Description: Beans in general are higher in protein than most other vegetables. They are often described by their shape or color. They are listed here separately due to the differences in the nutritive value.

NUTRIENTS:

Carbohydrates				40	gms
Proteins				16	gms
Fats				1	mg
	Cholesterol			0	mg
	Saturated			0.1	
Water				69	%
Fiber					gms
Minerals					
	Calcium			95	mg
	Iron			5.1	mg
	Magnesium				mg
Vitamins					
	A			0	I.U
	B1			0.27	mg
	B2			0.13	mg
	Niacin			1.3	mg
	B6				
	B12				mcg
	C			0	mg
	D				I.U
	E				I.U
	Folic acid				mcg
	K				mcg
Electrolytes					
	Sodium			13	mg
	Potassium			790	mg

BEANS, PINTO   **CAL: 265**

Type: Legume

Size: 1 cup cooked

Description: Beans in general are higher in protein than most other vegetables. They are often described by their shape or color. They are listed here separately due to the differences in the nutritive value. These are sometimes known as Indian Beans

NUTRIENTS:

Carbohydrates				49	gms
Proteins				15	gms
Fats				1	mg
	Cholesterol			0	mg
	Saturated			0.1	
Water				65	%
Fiber					gms
Minerals					
	Calcium			86	mg
	Iron			5.4	mg
	Magnesium				mg
Vitamins					
	A			tr	I.U
	B1			0.33	mg
	B2			0.16	mg
	Niacin			0.7	mg
	B6				
	B12				mcg
	C			0	mg
	D				I.U
	E				I.U
	Folic acid				mcg
	K				mcg
Electrolytes					
	Sodium			3	mg
	Potassium			882	mg

CAL: 230   **BEANS, RED KIDNEY**

Type: LEGUME

Size: 1 cup canned, cooked, solids and liquids

Description: Beans in general, are higher in protein than most other vegetables. They are frequently described by their shape or color. The Red Kidney is called this way because some believe it is the same shape as a kidney.

Carbohydrates				42	gms
Proteins				15	gms
Fats				1	mg
	Cholesterol			0	mg
	Saturated			0.1	
Water				76	%
Fiber					gms
Minerals					
	Calcium			74	mg
	Iron			4.6	mg
	Magnesium				mg
Vitamins					
	A			10	I.U
	B1			0.13	mg
	B2			0.10	mg
	Niacin			1.5	mg
	B6				
	B12				mcg
	C			0	mg
	D				I.U
	E				I.U
	Folic acid				mcg
	K				mcg
Electrolytes					
	Sodium			968	mg
	Potassium			673	mg

BEANS, SNAP   **CAL: 45**

Type: Vegetable

Size: 1 cup cooked, and drained

Description: There are two types of this Lily of the Valley member; green and white. The white has a thicker stem and only the tip is edible whereas all of the stem of the green is eaten.

NUTRIENTS:

Carbohydrates				10	gms
Proteins				2	gms
Fats				tr	mg
	Cholesterol			0	mg
	Saturated			0.1	
Water				89	%
Fiber					gms
Minerals					
	Calcium			58	mg
	Iron			1.6	mg
	Magnesium				mg
Vitamins					
	A			830	I.U
	B1			0.09	mg
	B2			0.12	mg
	Niacin			0.8	mg
	B6				
	B12				mcg
	C			12	mg
	D				I.U
	E				I.U
	Folic acid				mcg
	K				mcg
Electrolytes					
	Sodium			4	mg
	Potassium			374	mg

Type: Vegetable

Size: 1 cup cooked and drained

Description: These are considered root vegetables and are red in color. The leaves are also eaten and considered to be nutritious on their own. Both the root and leaf require careful cooking to retain their nutritive value. There is also a white beet grown mainly as a source of sugar.

NUTRIENTS:

Carbohydrates				8	gms
Proteins				4	gms
Fats				tr	mg
	Cholesterol			0	mg
	Saturated			tr	
Water				89	%
Fiber					gms
Minerals					
	Calcium			164	mg
	Iron			2.7	mg
	Magnesium				mg
Vitamins					
	A			7,340	I.U
	B1			0.17	mg
	B2			0.42	mg
	Niacin			0.7	mg
	B6				
	B12				mcg
	C			36	mg
	D				I.U
	E				I.U
	Folic acid				mcg
	K				mcg
Electrolytes					
	Sodium			347	mg
	Potassium			1,390	mg

Type: Vegetable

Size: 1 cup cooked, drained, diced or sliced

Description: These are considered root vegetables and are red in color. The leaves are also eaten and considered to be nutritious on their own. Both the root and leaf require careful cooking to retain their nutritive value. There is also a white beet grown mainly as a source of sugar

NUTRIENTS:

Carbohydrates				11	gms
Proteins				2	gms
Fats				tr	mg
	Cholesterol			0	mg
	Saturated			tr	
Water				91	%
Fiber					gms
Minerals					
	Calcium			19	mg
	Iron			1.1	mg
	Magnesium				mg
Vitamins					
	A			20	I.U
	B1			2	mg
	B2			0.05	mg
	Niacin			0.5	mg
	B6				
	B12				mcg
	C			9	mg
	D				I.U
	E				I.U
	Folic acid				mcg
	K				mcg
Electrolytes					
	Sodium			83	mg
	Potassium			530	mg

Type: Fruit

Size: 1 cup

Description: These grow on a bush and are usually harvested in the summer months. They are used in beverages such as juices, wines and cordials and as jams or preserves in addition to being eaten raw.

NUTRIENTS:

Carbohydrates				18	gms
Proteins				1	gms
Fats				1	mg
	Cholesterol			0	mg
	Saturated			0.2	
Water				86	%
Fiber				5.9	gms
Minerals					
	Calcium			46	mg
	Iron			0.8	mg
	Magnesium			2.9	mg
Vitamins					
	A			240	I.U
	B1			0.04	mg
	B2			0.11	mg
	Niacin			0.6	mg
	B6			0.089	
	B12			0	mcg
	C			30	mg
	D				I.U
	E				I.U
	Folic acid				mcg
	K				mcg
Electrolytes					
	Sodium			tr	mg
	Potassium			282	mg

BERRIES, BLUE   **CAL: 80**

Type: Fruit

Size: 1 cup

Description: This is a small round berry whose name describes its color.. There are similar berries grown in other parts of the world, which look alike, and are sometimes all called blueberries, buckleberries, bilberries and whortleberries. They are eaten raw or cooked in pies, pastries, jams and preserves.

NUTRIENTS:

Carbohydrates				18	gms
Proteins				1	gms
Fats				1	mg
	Cholesterol			0	mg
	Saturated			tr	
Water				85	%
Fiber				1.88	gms
Minerals					
	Calcium			9	mg
	Iron			0.2	mg
	Magnesium			7	mg
Vitamins					
	A			150	I.U
	B1			0.07	mg
	B2			0.07	mg
	Niacin			0.5	mg
	B6			0.52	
	B12			0	mcg
	C			19	mg
	D				I.U
	E				I.U
	Folic acid			9.3	mcg
	K				mcg
Electrolytes					
	Sodium			9	mg
	Potassium			129	mg

Type: Fruit

Size: 1 cup raw

Description: These are small purplish black berries that grow in umbrella shaped cluster with long red stems on shrubs. The fruit is quite sweet and the berries are most often used in combination with other berries in pies. The juice is common in wine.

NUTRIENTS:

Carbohydrates				26.7	gms
Proteins				95	gms
Fats				74	mg
	Cholesterol			0	mg
	Saturated				
Water				79	%
Fiber				10.15	gms
Minerals					
	Calcium			55	mg
	Iron			2.32	mg
	Magnesium			56	mg
Vitamins					
	A			870	I.U
	B1			102	mg
	B2			0.87	mg
	Niacin			725	mg
	B6			33	
	B12			0	mcg
	C			52	mg
	D				I.U
	E				I.U
	Folic acid				mcg
	K				mcg
Electrolytes					
	Sodium			4	mg
	Potassium			406	mg

BERRIES GOOSE   **CAL: 67**

Type: Fruit
Size: 1cup, cooked

Description: Although the fruit of this thorny bush is often found growing wild, the cultivated plant produces a larger and less acid berry. It is quite sour in taste and is rarely eaten raw but are used in pies, jams etc. These fruit belong to the same family as currants but have a thorny stem. They do poorly in areas where the summers are hot.

NUTRIENTS:

Carbohydrates				15.27	gms
Proteins				1.32	gms
Fats				87	mg
	Cholesterol			0	mg
	Saturated			.05	
Water				87	%
Fiber				2.85	gms
Minerals					
	Calcium			38	mg
	Iron			47	mg
	Magnesium			15	mg
Vitamins					
	A			435	I.U
	B1			.06	mg
	B2			.045	mg
	Niacin			.45	mg
	B6			12	
	B12			0	mcg
	C			41.6	mg
	D				I.U
	E				I.U
	Folic acid				mcg
	K				
Electrolytes					
	Sodium			1	mg
	Potassium			297	mg

Type: Fruit

Size: 10 raw

Description: Generally this is the fruit of a large tree, however, some varieties are found in shrubs. They appear in several colors, black, dark red and white. The black and the red are eaten alone or in combination, fresh. The white is considered too sweet for most palates and is rarely eaten raw. Wine is a common product from this fruit. Of note, the leaves used to be food for silk worms.

NUTRIENTS:

Carbohydrates				1.47	gms
Proteins				22	gms
Fats				0.6	mg
	Cholesterol				mg
	Saturated				
Water				86	%
Fiber				0.14	gms
Minerals					
	Calcium			6	mg
	Iron			0.28	mg
	Magnesium			3	mg
Vitamins					
	A			4	I.U
	B1			0	mg
	B2			0.034	mg
	Niacin			0.1	mg
	B6				
	B12			0	mcg
	C			5.5	mg
	D				I.U
	E				I.U
	Folic acid				mcg
	K				mcg
Electrolytes					
	Sodium			2	mg
	Potassium			29	mg

BLACK EYED PEAS   **CAL: 190**

Type: Legume

Size: 1 cup cooked

Description: Although these carry the word peas in the name, They are actually a legume and should be considered more correctly, a bean. Small, round, white/beige in color, they are distinctive for the dark almost black centers. This type of bean is frequently associated with southern United States cuisine and is a favorite eaten with corn bread. For some southerners, it is a must item as the first meal of the New Year for bringing good luck.

NUTRIENTS:

Carbohydrates				35	gms
Proteins				13	gms
Fats				1	mg
	Cholesterol			0	mg
	Saturated			9.2	
Water				80	%
Fiber					gms
Minerals					
	Calcium			43	mg
	Iron			3.3	mg
	Magnesium				mg
Vitamins					
	A			30	I.U
	B1			0.40	mg
	B2			0.10	mg
	Niacin			1.0	mg
	B6				
	B12				mcg
	C			0	mg
	D				I.U
	E				I.U
	Folic acid				mcg
	K				mcg
Electrolytes					
	Sodium			20	mg
	Potassium			573	mg

Type: Seed

Size: 1 oz shelled

Description: These hard shelled nuts are dark brown in color with length wise ridges. The meat of the nut is white in color. They are fairly popular nuts occupying a prominent place in most mixtures of "fancy" nuts. These nuts keep fairly well in the shell. These have also been called cream nut, butter nut, or shoe nut.

NUTRIENTS:

Carbohydrates				4	gms
Proteins				4	gms
Fats				1	mg
	Cholesterol			0	mg
	Saturated			1.2	
Water				3	%
Fiber					gms
Minerals					
	Calcium			50	mg
	Iron			1.0	mg
	Magnesium				mg
Vitamins					
	A			tr	I.U
	B1			0.28	mg
	B2			0.03	mg
	Niacin			0.5	mg
	B6				
	B12				mcg
	C			tr	
	D				I.U
	E				I.U
	Folic acid				mcg
	K				mcg
Electrolytes					
	Sodium			1	mg
	Potassium			170	mg

BREADFRUIT

Type: Fruit

Size: 1 cup raw

Description: This fruit, which grows four to seven inches in diameter, comes from a tropical tree found commonly in the South Pacific Islands. It is similar in taste and flavor to sweet potatoes. It is sliced, dried and than ground into flour and used in baking.

NUTRIENTS:

Carbohydrates				59.7	gms
Proteins				2.35	gms
Fats				.51	mg
	Cholesterol			0	mg
	Saturated				
Water				71	%
Fiber				3.25	gms
Minerals					
	Calcium			38	mg
	Iron			1.19	mg
	Magnesium			56	mg
Vitamins					
	A			88	I.U
	B1			.24	mg
	B2			.07	mg
	Niacin			2.0	mg
	B6				
	B12			0	mcg
	C			64	mg
	D				I.U
	E				I.U
	Folic acid				mcg
	K				mcg
Electrolytes					
	Sodium			4	mg
	Potassium			1,077	mg

Type: Vegetable

Size: 1 cup cooked and drained, cut in ½ inch spears

Description: Some think that this cabbage family member was the original form of cauliflower. The edible portion grows at the head of a stalk in a manner similar to the cauliflower. Whereas the cauliflower is white in color the broccoli clusters are deep green with the leaves and stems a lighter yellowish green. The vegetable can be eaten raw but many prefer it steamed. The floweretts are possibly more popular for eating but the stalks are often peeled and steamed with sauces.

NUTRIENTS:

Carbohydrates				8	gms
Proteins				5	gms
Fats				tr	mg
	Cholesterol			0	mg
	Saturated			0.1	
Water				90	%
Fiber				1.7	gms
Minerals					
	Calcium			72	mg
	Iron			1.8	mg
	Magnesium			38	mg
Vitamins					
	A			17	I.U
	B1			0.13	mg
	B2			0.32	mg
	Niacin			1.2	mg
	B6			.22	
	B12			0	mcg
	C			97	mg
	D				I.U
	E				I.U
	Folic acid			78	mcg
	K			220	mcg
Electrolytes					
	Sodium			17	mg
	Potassium			253	mg

BRUSSELS SPROUTS   CAL: 38

Type: Legume

Size: 1 cup cooked

Description: Some people think of these as miniature cabbages. They grown along the stalk of the plant. After cooking, they tend to have a more dominant flavor than others in the cabbage family.

NUTRIENTS:

Carbohydrates				13	gms
Proteins				4	gms
Fats				1	mg
	Cholesterol			0	mg
	Saturated			0.2	
Water				87	%
Fiber				1.3	gms
Minerals					
	Calcium			56	mg
	Iron			1.9	mg
	Magnesium			20	mg
Vitamins					
	A			1,110	I.U
	B1			0.17	mg
	B2			0.12	mg
	Niacin			0.9	mg
	B6			.18	
	B12			0	mcg
	C			96	mg
	D				I.U
	E				I.U
	Folic acid			54	mcg
	K			219	mcg
Electrolytes					
	Sodium			33	mg
	Potassium			491	mg

Type: Vegetable

Size: 1 cup rae, shredded

Description: This leafy vegetable has many varieties and includes several other vegetables in its family. The raw, green variety is most nutritious and holds its own even when cooked. The leaf of this vegetable contains sulfur which when cooked forms hydrogen sulfide. The product is thought to be the source of the odor given to cooked cabbage, particularly if cooked for a long time.

NUTRIENTS:

Carbohydrates				4	gms
Proteins				1	gms
Fats				tr	mg
	Cholesterol			0	mg
	Saturated			tr	
Water				93	%
Fiber					gms
Minerals					
	Calcium			33	mg
	Iron			0.4	mg
	Magnesium				mg
Vitamins					
	A			90	I.U
	B1			0.04	mg
	B2			0.02	mg
	Niacin			0.2	mg
	B6				
	B12				mcg
	C			33	mg
	D				I.U
	E				I.U
	Folic acid				mcg
	K				mcg
Electrolytes					
	Sodium			13	mg
	Potassium			172	mg

Type: Vegetable

Size: 1 cup cooked, drained

Description: This is the form of the cabbage family that is commonly used in Chinese cooking. It differs in appearance from the common green cabbage in that instead of a compact round ball of consistent light green color, it is an elongated compaction of leaves which go from white in color at the base to green on the leaf ends.

NUTRIENTS:

Carbohydrates				3	gms
Proteins				3	gms
Fats				tr	mg
	Cholesterol			0	mg
	Saturated			tr	
Water				96	%
Fiber					gms
Minerals					
	Calcium			156	mg
	Iron			1.8	mg
	Magnesium				mg
Vitamins					
	A			4,370	I.U
	B1			0.05	mg
	B2			0.11	mg
	Niacin			0.7	mg
	B6				
	B12				mcg
	C			44	mg
	D				I.U
	E				I.U
	Folic acid				mcg
	K			164	mcg
Electrolytes					
	Sodium			58	mg
	Potassium			631	mg

CAL: 20   **CABBAGE, RED**

Type: Vegetable

Size: 1 cup raw. Shredded

Description: Another member of the cabbage family that is distinguished by its red and purplish color. It is thought to be an early fall variety. It is consumed raw and cooked. Like other members of the cabbage family, it should be cooked with only enough water to cover the leaves and only until the leaves are tender. Over cooking decreases the appearance and palatability.

NUTRIENTS:

Carbohydrates				4	gms
Proteins				1	gms
Fats				tr	mg
	Cholesterol			0	mg
	Saturated			tr	
Water				92	%
Fiber					gms
Minerals					
	Calcium			36	mg
	Iron			0.3	mg
	Magnesium				mg
Vitamins					
	A			30	I.U
	B1			0.04	mg
	B2			0.02	mg
	Niacin			0.2	mg
	B6				
	B12				mcg
	C			40	mg
	D				I.U
	E				I.U
	Folic acid				mcg
	K				mcg
Electrolytes					
	Sodium			8	mg
	Potassium			144	mg

CANTALOUPE   CAL:95

Type: Fruit
Size: ½ of a 5 inch diameter size

Description: One of several types of melons that belong to the group which are botanically mask melons. The skins are beige/brown in color when ripe but are frequently seen in the market somewhat greenish in color. These have not fully matured and generally are not ripe. If placed in a brown paper bag at room temperature, they continue to ripen. They are almost never cooked but eaten raw, alone or in various other dishes.

NUTRIENTS:

Carbohydrates				22	gms
Proteins				2	gms
Fats				1	mg
	Cholesterol			0	mg
	Saturated			0.1	
Water				90	%
Fiber				.97	gms
Minerals					
	Calcium			29	mg
	Iron			0.6	mg
	Magnesium			28	mg
Vitamins					
	A			8,610	I.U
	B1			0.2	mg
	B2			0.06	mg
	Niacin			1.5	mg
	B6			.31	
	B12			0	mcg
	C			113	mg
	D				I.U
	E				I.U
	Folic acid			46.5	mcg
	K				
Electrolytes					
	Sodium			24	mg
	Potassium			825	mg

CARAMBOLA

Type: Fruit
Size: 1 raw

Description: This is an oval shaped fruit. It has a thin smooth skin and is fragrant in odor. Eaten either raw or cooked, it has a taste that ranges from acid to sweet. The tree is known in East India.

NUTRIENTS:

Carbohydrates				9.9	gms
Proteins				0.69	gms
Fats				0.44	mg
	Cholesterol			0	mg
	Saturated				
Water				90	%
Fiber				1.17	gms
Minerals					
	Calcium			6	mg
	Iron			0.33	mg
	Magnesium			12	mg
Vitamins					
	A			626	I.U
	B1			0.04	mg
	B2			0.03	mg
	Niacin			0.55	mg
	B6				
	B12			0	mcg
	C			27	mg
	D				I.U
	E				I.U
	Folic acid				mcg
	K				
Electrolytes					
	Sodium			2	mg
	Potassium			207	mg

Type: Vegetable

Size: 1 1 raw approximately 7 ½ inch long

Description: The carrot is considered a root vegetable. It is consumed both raw and in cooked form. The nutritive value decreases as it gets older and with cooking the amount of water.

NUTRIENTS:

Carbohydrates				7	gms
Proteins				1	gms
Fats				tr	mg
	Cholesterol			0	mg
	Saturated			tr	
Water				88	%
Fiber					gms
Minerals					
	Calcium			19	mg
	Iron			0.4	mg
	Magnesium			2	mg
Vitamins					
	A			20,250	I.U
	B1			0.07	mg
	B2			0.04	mg
	Niacin			0.7	mg
	B6			.012	
	B12			0	mcg
	C			7	mg
	D				I.U
	E				I.U
	Folic acid			5	mcg
	K			16	mcg
Electrolytes					
	Sodium			25	mg
	Potassium			233	mg

Type: Seed

Size: 1 oz ,dry roasted, salted

Description: The flavor of this kidney shaped nut resembles that of an almond. These nuts are found encased in a hard shell. Some people are sensitive to a substance found in the shell and can develop blisters. Roasting appears to remove this problem.

NUTRIENTS:

Carbohydrates				9	gms
Proteins				4	gms
Fats				13	mg
	Cholesterol			0	mg
	Saturated			2.6	
Water				2	%
Fiber					gms
Minerals					
	Calcium			13	mg
	Iron			1.7	mg
	Magnesium				mg
Vitamins					
	A			0	I.U
	B1			0.06	mg
	B2			0.06	mg
	Niacin			0.4	mg
	B6				
	B12				mcg
	C			0	mg
	D				I.U
	E				I.U
	Folic acid				mcg
	K			20	mcg
Electrolytes					
	Sodium			181	mg
	Potassium			160	mg

CAULIFLOWER

Type: Vegetable

Size: 1 cup raw

Description: Another member of the cabbage family. It is similar in appearance to the Broccoli head with the difference one of color and the number of flowerets. The cauliflower is one compact head as a unique entity and is white in color. Some consider the flavor more mild than that of other members of this family.

NUTRIENTS:

Carbohydrates				5	gms
Proteins				2	gms
Fats				tr	mg
	Cholesterol			0	mg
	Saturated			tr	
Water				92	%
Fiber					gms
Minerals					
	Calcium			29	mg
	Iron			0.6	mg
	Magnesium				mg
Vitamins					
	A			20	I.U
	B1			0.08	mg
	B2			0.06	mg
	Niacin			0.6	mg
	B6				
	B12				mcg
	C			72	mg
	D				I.U
	E				I.U
	Folic acid				mcg
	K				mcg
Electrolytes					
	Sodium			15	mg
	Potassium			355	mg

CELERY

Type: Legume

Size: 1 stalk, 8 inches long, raw

Description: The celery stalk is one of the few vegetables that is utilized in almost its entirety. From the leaves to the stalks themselves, it is eaten raw or cooked in any number of ways. It is low in calories but also low in overall nutritive value. It is high in cellulose which provides bulk in the diet.

NUTRIENTS:

Carbohydrates				1	gms
Proteins				tr	gms
Fats				tr	mg
	Cholesterol			0	mg
	Saturated			tr	
Water				95	%
Fiber				.32	gms
Minerals					
	Calcium			14	mg
	Iron			0.2	mg
	Magnesium			4	mg
Vitamins					
	A			0.01	I.U
	B1			0.01	mg
	B2			0.1	mg
	Niacin			0.18	mg
	B6			0	
	B12			3	mcg
	C				mg
	D				I.U
	E				I.U
	Folic acid			11	mcg
	K				mcg
Electrolytes					
	Sodium			35	mg
	Potassium			114	mg

CHERRIES   **CAL: 50**

Type: Fruit

Size: 10 raw

Description: A small around fruit that was at one time considered a summer fruit. It is no longer. It can be found in most markets in the United States at all times of the year. There are supposedly around 250 different varieties. These are eaten raw or cooked. A favorite method of presentation is the cherry pie.

NUTRIENTS:

Carbohydrates				11	gms
Proteins				1	gms
Fats				1	mg
	Cholesterol			0	mg
	Saturated			0.1	
Water				81	%
Fiber				0.21	gms
Minerals					
	Calcium			0	mg
	Iron			0.3	mg
	Magnesium			9	mg
Vitamins					
	A			150	I.U
	B1			0.03	mg
	B2			0.04	mg
	Niacin			0.3	mg
	B6			0.045	
	B12			0	mcg
	C			5	mg
	D				I.U
	E				I.U
	Folic acid			7.7	mcg
	K				mcg
Electrolytes					
	Sodium			tr	mg
	Potassium			152	mg

Type: Seed

Size: 1 cup roasted, shelled (European)

Description: This nut grows on a tree and belongs to the beech family. Europe and America are common locations it. The nuts are usually roasted.

NUTRIENTS:

Carbohydrates				76	gms
Proteins				5	gms
Fats				3	mg
	Cholesterol			0	mg
	Saturated			0.6	
Water				40	%
Fiber					gms
Minerals					
	Calcium			41	mg
	Iron			1.3	mg
	Magnesium				mg
Vitamins					
	A			30	I.U
	B1			0.35	mg
	B2			0.25	mg
	Niacin			1.9	mg
	B6				
	B12				mcg
	C			37	mg
	D				I.U
	E				I.U
	Folic acid				mcg
	K				mcg
Electrolytes					
	Sodium			3	mg
	Potassium			847	mg

COCONUT   **CAL: 285**

Type: Nut

Size: 1 cup raw, shredded or grated

Description: This tree is found commonly in tropical countries. The edible portion is usually the white meat which comes encased within a hard brown shell. Natives of the countries where it is grown often eat the meat raw. In many of the countries to which it is exported, it is often dried, shredded with sugar and salt is added. The milk of the nut is often used in cooking. Dried coconut meat is called copra. The extracted oil is utilized in many products and is not limited to foods.

NUTRIENTS:

Carbohydrates				12	gms
Proteins				3	gms
Fats				15	mg
	Cholesterol			0	mg
	Saturated			23.8	
Water				47	%
Fiber					gms
Minerals					
	Calcium			11	mg
	Iron			1.9	mg
	Magnesium				mg
Vitamins					
	A			0	I.U
	B1			0.05	mg
	B2			0.02	mg
	Niacin			0.4	mg
	B6				
	B12				mcg
	C			3	mg
	D				I.U
	E				I.U
	Folic acid				mcg
	K				mcg
Electrolytes					
	Sodium			16	mg
	Potassium			285	mg

Type: Vegetable

Size: 1 cup kernels

Description: A very important vegetable in the United States. It is grown for both human and animal consumption. It provides the basis for many products. It is eaten directly from the ear., The kernels are sometimes separated and are made into meal, cereal, oil syrup etc. In France at one time, it was only used as animal feed. It is said that the Indians named this maize, although there may be a difference in the variety. There are many varieties. Americans are very familiar with the variety that is popped.

NUTRIENTS:

Carbohydrates				34	gms
Proteins				5	gms
Fats				tr	mg
	Cholesterol			0	mg
	Saturated			tr	
Water				73	%
Fiber					gms
Minerals					
	Calcium			3	mg
	Iron			0.5	mg
	Magnesium				mg
Vitamins					
	A			410	I.U
	B1			0.11	mg
	B2			0.12	mg
	Niacin			2.1	mg
	B6				
	B12				mcg
	C			4	mg
	D				I.U
	E				I.U
	Folic acid				mcg
	K				mcg
Electrolytes					
	Sodium			8	mg
	Potassium			229	mg

CRANBERRY SAUCE   **CAL: 420**

Type: Fruit

Size: 1 cup cooked, canned and sweetened

Description: A cooked sauce made from this deep and red berry with sugar added. It is found in the markets in a canned and jellied form most frequently but the raw berries can also be purchased. They are thought to have a substance, which becomes hippuric acid and is excreted in the urine. It is a common finding on the American menu at Christmas and Thanksgiving time

NUTRIENTS:

Carbohydrates				108	gms
Proteins				1	gms
Fats				tr	mg
	Cholesterol			0	mg
	Saturated			tr	
Water				61	%
Fiber				0.83	gms
Minerals					
	Calcium			11	mg
	Iron			0.6	mg
	Magnesium			8	mg
Vitamins					
	A			60	I.U
	B1			0.04	mg
	B2			0.06	mg
	Niacin			0.3	mg
	B6			0.039	
	B12			0	mcg
	C			6	mg
	D				I.U
	E				I.U
	Folic acid				mcg
	K				mcg
Electrolytes					
	Sodium			80	mg
	Potassium			72	mg

Type: Vegetable

Size: 6 large slices (splices 1/8 th inch thick, 2 and 1/8th inch in diameter)

Description: This member of the gourd family is cylindrical in shape with a dark green outer covering and pale green flesh. Although it is almost always eaten raw, many are preserved and pickled. Some believe that the plant originated in India.

NUTRIENTS:

Carbohydrates				1	gms
Proteins				tr	gms
Fats				tr	mg
	Cholesterol			0	mg
	Saturated			tr	
Water				96	%
Fiber					gms
Minerals					
	Calcium			4	mg
	Iron			0.1	mg
	Magnesium				mg
Vitamins					
	A			10	I.U
	B1			0.01	mg
	B2			0.1	mg
	Niacin				mg
	B6				
	B12				mcg
	C			1	mg
	D				I.U
	E				I.U
	Folic acid				mcg
	K				mcg
Electrolytes					
	Sodium			1	mg
	Potassium			42	mg

DATES   **CAL: 230**

Type: Fruit

Size: 10 pitted and whole

Description: Sometimes these are also classified as a confection. California and Arizona are common sites of growth. They are eaten raw and often used in baked goods. Some think that the plant was originally introduced into the southwestern United States by Spanish missionaries.

NUTRIENTS:

Carbohydrates				61	gms
Proteins				2	gms
Fats				tr	mg
	Cholesterol			0	mg
	Saturated			0.1	
Water				23	%
Fiber				1.83	gms
Minerals					
	Calcium			27	mg
	Iron			1.0	mg
	Magnesium			29	mg
Vitamins					
	A			40	I.U
	B1			0.07	mg
	B2			0.08	mg
	Niacin			1.8	mg
	B6			.34	
	B12			0	mcg
	C			0	mg
	D				I.U
	E				I.U
	Folic acid			22.4	mcg
	K				mcg
Electrolytes					
	Sodium			2	mg
	Potassium			541	mg

Type: Legume

Size: 1cup dried, cooked, drained

Description: These are also known as soybeans. They are considered by many as a very nutritious food, They have a high protein composition which is similar to that of the animal sources. The beans are eaten both fresh and cooked. Cheeses, milk, flour and a sauce are some of he most common usages of these legumes.

NUTRIENTS:

Carbohydrates				19	gms
Proteins				20	gms
Fats				10	mg
	Cholesterol			0	mg
	Saturated			1.3	
Water				71	%
Fiber					gms
Minerals					
	Calcium			131	mg
	Iron			4.9	mg
	Magnesium				mg
Vitamins					
	A			50	I.U
	B1			0.38	mg
	B2			0.16	mg
	Niacin			1.1	mg
	B6				
	B12				mcg
	C				mg
	D				I.U
	E				I.U
	Folic acid				mcg
	K			86	mcg
Electrolytes					
	Sodium			4	mg
	Potassium			972	mg

EGGPLANT   **CAL: 25**

Type: Fruit

Size: 1 cup cooked

Description: Most people think of this as a vegetable but botanically speaking it is a fruit. It is not sweet in taste as are many fruits. The type found in the United States most often is egg shaped and hence the name. The skin is purplish in color and smooth in texture. The lighter weights tend to be more flavorful while the heavier ones tend to have more seeds and a bitter taste. This fruit is prepared most often by boiling, baking or frying.

NUTRIENTS:

Carbohydrates				7	gms
Proteins				tr	gms
Fats				tr	mg
	Cholesterol			0	mg
	Saturated			tr	
Water				92	%
Fiber					gms
Minerals					
	Calcium			6	mg
	Iron			0.3	mg
	Magnesium				mg
Vitamins					
	A			60	I.U
	B1			0.07	mg
	B2			0.02	mg
	Niacin			0.6	mg
	B6				
	B12				mcg
	C			1	mg
	D				I.U
	E				I.U
	Folic acid				mcg
	K				
Electrolytes					
	Sodium			3	mg
	Potassium			238	mg

Type: Vegetable

Size: 1 cup raw

Description: A leafy vegetable that is used most often in salads. Its leaves are an off white in color and are tightly wrapped in an oval shape. The leaves have a bitter taste..

NUTRIENTS:

Carbohydrates				6	gms
Proteins				1	gms
Fats				tr	mg
	Cholesterol			0	mg
	Saturated			tr	
Water				94	%
Fiber					gms
Minerals					
	Calcium			26	mg
	Iron			0.4	mg
	Magnesium				mg
Vitamins					
	A			1,030	I.U
	B1			0.04	mg
	B2			0.04	mg
	Niacin			0.2	mg
	B6				
	B12				mcg
	C			3	mg
	D				I.U
	E				I.U
	Folic acid				mcg
	K			116	mcg
Electrolytes					
	Sodium			11	mg
	Potassium			157	mg

Type: Fruit

Size: 10 dried

Description: Once these somewhat pear shaped fruits were thought of as Oriental fruit. They were thought to be an emblem of prosperity and often employed in many religious ceremonies. The ripe fruit is considered fragile and does not take well to handling or long storage. It is most often found in the dried form.

NUTRIENTS:

Carbohydrates				122	gms
Proteins				6	gms
Fats				2	mg
	Cholesterol			0	mg
	Saturated			0.4	
Water				28	%
Fiber				8.97	gms
Minerals					
	Calcium			269	mg
	Iron			4.20	mg
	Magnesium			111	mg
Vitamins					
	A			250	I.U
	B1			0.13	mg
	B2			0.16	mg
	Niacin			1.3	mg
	B6			.42	
	B12			0	mcg
	C			1	mg
	D				I.U
	E				I.U
	Folic acid			14.1	mcg
	K				mcg
Electrolytes					
	Sodium			21	mg
	Potassium			1,331	mg

FILBERTS

Type: Seed

Size: 1 oz chopped

Description: These nuts are often known also as hazelnuts or cobnuts. They grow on bushes or clusters and come in several sizes and shapes. The Filbert is often larger in size than the hazelnut but all taste similarly. They are a common ingredient in nut breads and cakes.

NUTRIENTS:

Carbohydrates				4	gms
Proteins				4	gms
Fats				18	mg
	Cholesterol			0	mg
	Saturated			1.3	
Water				5	%
Fiber					gms
Minerals					
	Calcium			53	mg
	Iron			0.9	mg
	Magnesium				mg
Vitamins					
	A			20	I.U
	B1			0.14	mg
	B2			0.03	mg
	Niacin			0.3	mg
	B6				
	B12				mcg
	C			tr	mg
	D				I.U
	E				I.U
	Folic acid				mcg
	K				mcg
Electrolytes					
	Sodium			1	mg
	Potassium			126	mg

GRAPEFRUIT   **CAL: 40**

Type: Fruit

Size: ½ raw white

Description: California, Texas, and Florida have been traditionally the major growers of this member of the citrus family.. When choosing for eating, the heavier ones for the size are frequently the better pick, They are thought to be descended from the Dutch fruit called pompelmoes even though it is considered mainly an American product. In America some call it pomelo and the French word for grapefruit is pamplemouse.

NUTRIENTS:

Carbohydrates				10	gms
Proteins				tr	gms
Fats				tr	mg
	Cholesterol			tr	mg
	Saturated			tr	
Water				91	%
Fiber				.24	gms
Minerals					
	Calcium			14	mg
	Iron			0.1	mg
	Magnesium			0	mg
Vitamins					
	A			14	I.U
	B1			0.04	mg
	B2			0.02	mg
	Niacin			0.3	mg
	B6			.05	
	B12			0	mcg
	C			41	mg
	D				I.U
	E				I.U
	Folic acid			12.2	mcg
	K				mcg
Electrolytes					
	Sodium			tr	mg
	Potassium			167	mg

Type: Fruit

Size: 10 Thompson seedless

Description: These are small, usually round, sweet juicy fruits. The Thompson variety is seedless. They are eaten raw and also used in beverages, notably wine. They are grown in many places in the world. The Thompson variety is a very pale , almost whitish , green color. Recent research suggests that there may be something in the skin of red grapes that is cardio-protective.

NUTRIENTS:

Carbohydrates				9	gms
Proteins				tr	gms
Fats				tr	mg
	Cholesterol			0	mg
	Saturated			0.1	
Water				81	%
Fiber					gms
Minerals					
	Calcium			6	mg
	Iron			0.1	mg
	Magnesium				mg
Vitamins					
	A			40	I.U
	B1			0.05	mg
	B2			0.03	mg
	Niacin			0.2	mg
	B6				
	B12				mcg
	C			5	mg
	D				I.U
	E				I.U
	Folic acid				mcg
	K			28	mcg
Electrolytes					
	Sodium			1	mg
	Potassium			93	mg

GREENS, COLLARDS   **CAL: 25**

Type: Vegetable

Size: 1 cup cooked, drained

Description: These are the leaves that come from the collard plant. It is another member of the cabbage family. This cooked dish has traditionally been associated with southern cooking and is as common a menu item as spinach in other places. The flavor is distinctive and considered by some to be strong.

NUTRIENTS:

Carbohydrates				5	gms
Proteins				2	gms
Fats				tr	mg
	Cholesterol			0	mg
	Saturated			0.1	
Water				96	%
Fiber				.63	gms
Minerals					
	Calcium			148	mg
	Iron			0.810	mg
	Magnesium				mg
Vitamins					
	A			4,220	I.U
	B1			0.03	mg
	B2			0.08	mg
	Niacin			0.4	mg
	B6			.067	
	B12			0	mcg
	C			19	mg
	D				I.U
	E				I.U
	Folic acid			8	mcg
	K			836	mcg
Electrolytes					
	Sodium			36	mg
	Potassium			177	mg

Type: Vegetable

Size: 1 cup cooked, drained

Description: Very common as a food product. These can be found wild but are specifically cultivated for marketing. The most tender of the leaves are those that have not yet flowered. Once the leaves have blossomed, the taste changes somewhat and is thought to be bitterer. They are consumed raw and cooked.

NUTRIENTS:

Carbohydrates				7	gms
Proteins				2	gms
Fats				tr	mg
	Cholesterol			0	mg
	Saturated			tr	
Water				90	%
Fiber					gms
Minerals					
	Calcium			147	mg
	Iron			0.3	mg
	Magnesium				mg
Vitamins					
	A			12,290	I.U
	B1			0.14	mg
	B2			0.18	mg
	Niacin			0.5	mg
	B6				
	B12				mcg
	C			19	mg
	D				I.U
	E				I.U
	Folic acid				mcg
	K			778.4	mcg...?
					mcg
Electrolytes					
	Sodium			46	mg
	Potassium			244	mg

GREENS, MUSTARD   CAL: 20

Type: Vegetable

Size: 1 cup cooked, drained

Description: This group includes leaves that come from several species of the mustard plant. Because they have such ac acrid taste, the leaves are often mixed with milder greens in cooking.

NUTRIENTS:

Carbohydrates				6	gms
Proteins				3	gms
Fats				tr	mg
	Cholesterol			0	mg
	Saturated			tr	
Water				94	%
Fiber					gms
Minerals					
	Calcium			104	mg
	Iron			1.0	mg
	Magnesium				mg
Vitamins					
	A			4,240	I.U
	B1			0.06	mg
	B2			0.09	mg
	Niacin			0.6	mg
	B6				
	B12				mcg
	C			35	mg
	D				I.U
	E				I.U
	Folic acid				mcg
	K			420	mcg
Electrolytes					
	Sodium			22	mg
	Potassium			283	mg

CAL: 30   **GREENS TURNIP**

Type: Vegetable

Size: 1 cup cooked and diced

Description: The leaf from the turnip plant is often cooked as a vegetable. The greatest nutritive value appears to be vitamin A.

NUTRIENTS:

Carbohydrates				6	gms
Proteins				2	gms
Fats				tr	mg
	Cholesterol			0	mg
	Saturated			0.3	
Water				93	%
Fiber					gms
Minerals					
	Calcium			197	mg
	Iron			1.2	mg
	Magnesium				mg
Vitamins					
	A			7,920	I.U
	B1			0.06	mg
	B2			0.10	mg
	Niacin			0.6	mg
	B6				
	B12				mcg
	C			39	mg
	D				I.U
	E				I.U
	Folic acid				mcg
	K			570	mcg
Electrolytes					
	Sodium			42	mg
	Potassium			292	mg

GUAVAS   **CAL: 45**

Type: Fruit

Size: 1 fruit raw

Description: This fruit comes from a semi-tropical tree common in Florida and California. They appear in several shapes namely, round, oval and pear shaped. The flesh of the fruit is eaten raw or canned in jellies and can range from acrid to sweet in taste. They are thought to belong to the Myrtle F/family.

NUTRIENTS:

Carbohydrates				10.69	gms
Proteins				0.74	gms
Fats				54	mg
	Cholesterol			0	mg
	Saturated			0.15	
Water				77.5	%
Fiber				5.04	gms
Minerals					
	Calcium			18	mg
	Iron			0.28	mg
	Magnesium			9	mg
Vitamins					
	A			713	I.U
	B1			0.045	mg
	B2			0..045	mg
	Niacin			1.08	mg
	B6			0.129	
	B12			0	mcg
	C			165	mg
	D				I.U
	E				I.U
	Folic acid				mcg
	K				mcg
Electrolytes					
	Sodium			2	mg
	Potassium			256	mg

CAL: 45

Type: Fruit

Size: 1/10th of a 6 ½ inch diameter size

Description: One of several types of melons. The skin is a pale green , almost white color and is smooth to touch. The fruit inside is also greenish. In checking for ripeness,, the entire skin should be smooth, somewhat soft and very aromatic.

NUTRIENTS:

Carbohydrates				12	gms
Proteins				1	gms
Fats				tr	mg
	Cholesterol			0	mg
	Saturated			tr	
Water				90	%
Fiber				0.77	gms
Minerals					
	Calcium			8	mg
	Iron			0.1	mg
	Magnesium			9	mg
Vitamins					
	A			50	I.U
	B1			0.10	mg
	B2			0.02	mg
	Niacin			0.8	mg
	B6			0.7	
	B12			0	mcg
	C			32	mg
	D				I.U
	E				I.U
	Folic acid				mcg
	K				mcg
Electrolytes					
	Sodium			13	mg
	Potassium			350	mg

KALE   **CAL: 40**

Type: Vegetable

Size: 1 cup cooked, drained

Description: This is another member of the cabbage family but it does not form a head. There are many different types, which are distinguished by their leaves. These leaves vary from plain, wavy or curly. Shades of greens, reddish brown, and purple are seen in the leaves. Even though this is a member of the cabbage family, many people cook and serve kale as they do the other vegetable greens.

NUTRIENTS:

Carbohydrates				7	gms
Proteins				2	gms
Fats				1	mg
	Cholesterol			0	mg
	Saturated			0.1	
Water				91	%
Fiber					gms
Minerals					
	Calcium			94	mg
	Iron			1.2	mg
	Magnesium				mg
Vitamins					
	A			9,620	I.U
	B1			0.07	mg
	B2			0.09	mg
	Niacin			0.7	mg
	B6				
	B12				mcg
	C			53	mg
	D				I.U
	E				I.U
	Folic acid				mcg
	K			106.2	mcg
Electrolytes					
	Sodium			30	mg
	Potassium			296	mg

Type: Fruit

Size: 1 peeled, approximately 1/3rd of a pound

Description: A small fruit tending to a lightly tart flavor for the pulp inside. The skin is not usually eaten but the fruit is mostly consumed raw. It is frequently seen decorating tart pastries. Generally it is though to have been introduced into the American market from Australia.

NUTRIENTS:

Carbohydrates				11	gms
Proteins				tr	gms
Fats				tr	mg
	Cholesterol			0	mg
	Saturated			tr	
Water				83	%
Fiber				0.84	gms
Minerals					
	Calcium			20	mg
	Iron			0.3	mg
	Magnesium			2.3	mg
Vitamins					
	A			130	I.U
	B1			0.02	mg
	B2			0.04	mg
	Niacin			0.4	mg
	B6				
	B12				mcg
	C			74	mg
	D				I.U
	E				I.U
	Folic acid				mcg
	K				mcg
Electrolytes					
	Sodium			4	mg
	Potassium			252	mg

KOHLRABI

Type: Vegetable

Size: 1 cup cooked, drained

Description: This is a another member of the cabbage family. The edible portion is a thickened root portion that grows above the ground and looks similar to a turnip in shape. When it is prepared soon after it grows, it tends to have a flavor more delicate than the turnip. It is served both cold in salads and as a hot vegetable.

NUTRIENTS:

Carbohydrates				11	gms
Proteins				3	gms
Fats				tr	mg
	Cholesterol			0	mg
	Saturated			tr	
Water				90	%
Fiber					gms
Minerals					
	Calcium			41	mg
	Iron			0.7	mg
	Magnesium				mg
Vitamins					
	A			60	I.U
	B1			0.07	mg
	B2			0.03	mg
	Niacin			0.6	mg
	B6				
	B12				mcg
	C			89	mg
	D				I.U
	E				I.U
	Folic acid				mcg
	K				mcg
Electrolytes					
	Sodium			1	mg
	Potassium			561	mg

KUMQQUATS

Type: Fruit

Size: 1 fruit raw

Description: These fruits belong to the citrus family. They are small, bright orange in color and the rind or skin is sweet. The flesh is quite tart. Because of the contrast, the fruit is often cooked in heavy syrup and also made into jams and marmalades. When the fruit is eaten raw, it is the rind, which is the most popular part. Some devotees of the fruit suggest plopping the entire fruit in the mouth at once and chewing it "en-mass". They claim that it is the only way to really appreciate it eaten raw. It is thought to have originated in China but today is commonly found in the United States; in Southern California.

NUTRIENTS:

Carbohydrates				3.12	gms
Proteins				0.17	gms
Fats				0.02	mg
	Cholesterol			0	mg
	Saturated				
Water				75	%
Fiber				0.70	gms
Minerals					
	Calcium			8	mg
	Iron			0.07	mg
	Magnesium			2	mg
Vitamins					
	A			57	I.U
	B1			0.015	mg
	B2			0.019	mg
	Niacin			0.39	mg
	B6				
	B12				mcg
	C			7.1	mg
	D				I.U
	E				I.U
	Folic acid				mcg
	K				mcg
Electrolytes					
	Sodium			1	mg
	Potassium			37	mg

LEMON　　　　　　　　　　　　　　　　　　　　　　　　　**CAL: 15**

Type: Fruit

Size: 1 approximately ¼ of a pound

Description: A popular member of the citrus family. A quite hardy fruit that is used in beverages and cooking. Some think it compliments fish dishes well by counteracting the fatty taste. They are thought to have been introduced into Spain by the Arabs in the twelfth century.

NUTRIENTS:

Carbohydrates				5	gms
Proteins				1	gms
Fats				tr	mg
	Cholesterol			tr	mg
	Saturated			tr	
Water				89	%
Fiber					gms
Minerals					
	Calcium			15	mg
	Iron			0.3	mg
	Magnesium			13	mg
Vitamins					
	A			20	I.U
	B1			0.02	mg
	B2			0.01	mg
	Niacin			0.1	mg
	B6			0.12	
	B12				mcg
	C			31	mg
	D				I.U
	E				I.U
	Folic acid				mcg
	K				mcg
Electrolytes					
	Sodium			1	mg
	Potassium			80	mg

Type: Legume

Size: 1 cup dry, cooked

Description: These are thought to be the most nutrition of all legumes with the possible exception of the soy bean. Lentils are often served in stews and soups. To prepare them for eating they are soaked in water for several hours and the soaking water discarded. Afterward-fresh water is added and they are simmered slowly. There are claims that the Egyptian lentil was found on St. Peter's Island during the Bronze Age.

NUTRIENTS:

Carbohydrates				38	gms
Proteins				16	gms
Fats				1	mg
	Cholesterol			0	mg
	Saturated			0.1	
Water				72	%
Fiber					gms
Minerals					
	Calcium			50	mg
	Iron			4.2	mg
	Magnesium				mg
Vitamins					
	A			40	I.U
	B1			0.14	mg
	B2			0.12	mg
	Niacin			1.2	mg
	B6				
	B12				mcg
	C			0	mg
	D				I.U
	E				I.U
	Folic acid				mcg
	K				mcg
Electrolytes					
	Sodium			26	mg
	Potassium			498	mg

LETTUCE, BOSTON

Type: Vegetable

Size: 1 whole head

Description: This is only one of several forms of this vegetable. The main use for all of the lettuce plants is in salads. The Boston lettuce has a relatively small and loosely compacted head of leaves. The texture is coarser than the iceberg but tends to have straighter edges. Some people prefer to use this variety in sandwiches because the leaves tend to lay flatter and are easier to cut with a fork.

NUTRIENTS:

Carbohydrates				4	gms
Proteins				2	gms
Fats				tr	mg
	Cholesterol			0	mg
	Saturated			tr	
Water				96	%
Fiber					gms
Minerals					
	Calcium			52	mg
	Iron			0.5	mg
	Magnesium				mg
Vitamins					
	A			1,580	I.U
	B1			0.10	mg
	B2			0.10	mg
	Niacin			0.5	mg
	B6				
	B12				mcg
	C			1	mg
	D				I.U
	E				I.U
	Folic acid				mcg
	K				mcg
Electrolytes					
	Sodium			8	mg
	Potassium			419	mg

Type: Vegetable

Size: ¼ inch wedge, of a 6 inch in diameter, whole head

Description: This is only one of several forms of this vegetable. The main use for all of the lettuce plants is in salads. The iceberg lettuce has a compact head of pale green leaves. The texture is crisp and the edges tend to be a bit wavy. A reddish brown tinge along the edge of the outside leaves is a mark of true iceberg lettuce. An easy way to separate the leaves and obtain them unbroken is to core out the center root and place the head under cold water. The leaves will separate intact.

NUTRIENTS:

Carbohydrates				3	gms
Proteins				1	gms
Fats				tr	mg
	Cholesterol			0	mg
	Saturated			tr	
Water				96	%
Fiber					gms
Minerals					
	Calcium			26	mg
	Iron			0.7	mg
	Magnesium				mg
Vitamins					
	A			450	I.U
	B1			0.06	mg
	B2			0.04	mg
	Niacin			0.3	mg
	B6				
	B12				mcg
	C			5	mg
	D				I.U
	E				I.U
	Folic acid				mcg
	K			142	mcg
Electrolytes					
	Sodium			12	mg
	Potassium			213	mg

LETTUCE, ROMAINE   CAL: 10

Type: Vegetable

Size: 1 cup

Description: This is only one of several forms of this vegetable. The main use for all of the lettuce plants is in salads. The name given to this one of what are sometimes called the loose-leaf types is Romaine. As stated, the leaves are loosely packed, the shape is elongated with crinkly edges and the leaves have a heavy center rib, which renders a crunchy taste. Some find the taste more bitter than the iceberg.

NUTRIENTS:

Carbohydrates				2	gms
Proteins				10	gms
Fats				tr	mg
	Cholesterol			tr	mg
	Saturated			tr	
Water				94	%
Fiber					gms
Minerals					
	Calcium			38	mg
	Iron			0.8	mg
	Magnesium				mg
Vitamins					
	A			1,060	I.U
	B1			0.03	mg
	B2			0.04	mg
	Niacin			0.2	mg
	B6				
	B12				mcg
	C			10	mg
	D				I.U
	E				I.U
	Folic acid				mcg
	K			114	mcg
Electrolytes					
	Sodium			5	mg
	Potassium			148	mg

Type: Fruit

Size: 1 raw

Description: A citrus family member. This fruit contains more citric acid proportionately to its weight than other numbers. The sour flavor is quite aromatic and distinctive from the lemon. Fresh limes do not keep well and should be stored in a cool dry place.

NUTRIENTS:

Carbohydrates				7.06	gms
Proteins				0.47	gms
Fats				13	mg
	Cholesterol			0	mg
	Saturated			0.15	
Water				88	%
Fiber				34	gms
Minerals					
	Calcium			22	mg
	Iron			0.40	mg
	Magnesium				mg
Vitamins					
	A			7	I.U
	B1			0.02	mg
	B2			0.01	mg
	Niacin			1.34	mg
	B6			0.129	
	B12				mcg
	C			19.5	mg
	D				I.U
	E				I.U
	Folic acid			5.5	mcg
	K				mcg
Electrolytes					
	Sodium			1	mg
	Potassium			68	mg

MACADAMIA NUTS   CAL: 205

Type: Seed

Size: 1 oz roasted in oil, salted

Description: This nut is smooth and shiny on its coat and usually large. It has also been called the Queensland nut. It is thought to be native to Australia. It is most commonly associated with Hawaii. Most people outside of Hawaii are used to the salted, canned and roasted presentation.

NUTRIENTS:

Carbohydrates				4	gms
Proteins				2	gms
Fats				22	mg
	Cholesterol			0	mg
	Saturated			3.2	
Water				2	%
Fiber					gms
Minerals					
	Calcium			13	mg
	Iron			0.5	mg
	Magnesium				mg
Vitamins					
	A			tr	I.U
	B1			0.06	mg
	B2			0.03	mg
	Niacin			0.6	mg
	B6				
	B12				mcg
	C			0	mg
	D				I.U
	E				I.U
	Folic acid				mcg
	K				mcg
Electrolytes					
	Sodium			74	mg
	Potassium			93	mg

MANGO

Type: Fruit

Size: 1 approximately ¾ lb in weight

Description: These fruits are often thought of as tropical but are grown in many places in the United States and Mexico. Hawaii is a common source. They arrive in all shapes, sizes and to some extent gradations in colors. The interior has a very juicy pulp which has fibers that arise from the quite large seed. It does not hold up well for any length of time and is usually eaten raw as soon as cut.

NUTRIENTS:

Carbohydrates				35	gms
Proteins				1	gms
Fats				1	mg
	Cholesterol			0	mg
	Saturated			0.1	
Water				93	%
Fiber				1.73	gms
Minerals					
	Calcium			21	mg
	Iron			0.3	mg
	Magnesium			18	mg
Vitamins					
	A			8,060	I.U
	B1			0.12	mg
	B2			0.12	mg
	Niacin			1.2	mg
	B6			.28	
	B12				mcg
	C			57	mg
	D				I.U
	E				I.U
	Folic acid				mcg
	K				mcg
Electrolytes					
	Sodium			4	mg
	Potassium			323	mg

MELONS, CASABA   **CAL: 45**

Type: Fruit

Size: 1 cup of fruit, fresh and cubed

Description: Although all melons are grossly classified as either of the watermelon or muskmelon type, each of these broader groups have several varieties. The Casaba melon falls in the muskmelon group. It was named for Kassaba, a town near Smyrna. Casaba melons tend to be large in size and are naturally ready in late summer and early autumn. The rind is netted and golden in color. The flesh is firm, smooth textured and deep cream in color. It has a small seed cavity.

NUTRIENTS:

Carbohydrates				10.54	gms
Proteins				1.53	gms
Fats				0.17	mg
	Cholesterol			0	mg
	Saturated				
Water				92	%
Fiber				0.85	gms
Minerals					
	Calcium			9	mg
	Iron			0.68	mg
	Magnesium			14	mg
Vitamins					
	A			5	I.U
	B1			0.10	mg
	B2			0.034	mg
	Niacin			0.68	mg
	B6				
	B12				mcg
	C			27.2	mg
	D				I.U
	E				I.U
	Folic acid				mcg
	K				mcg
Electrolytes					
	Sodium			20	mg
	Potassium			357	mg

CAL: 20   **MUSHROOMS**

Type: Vegetable

Size: 1 cup raw, sliced or chopped

Description: These vegetables belong to the fungi family. There are many edible varieties but only individuals well versed in botanical knowledge of these plants are advised to attempt to harvest them wild. The non-edible ones can be deadly. These vegetables are highly perishable and lose their flavor in storage and overcooking. The sodium and potassium listed below will differ if the product is canned and drained.

NUTRIENTS:

Carbohydrates				3	gms
Proteins				1	gms
Fats				tr	mg
	Cholesterol			0	mg
	Saturated			tr	
Water				92	%
Fiber					gms
Minerals					
	Calcium			9	mg
	Iron			2.7	mg
	Magnesium				mg
Vitamins					
	A			0	I.U
	B1			0.07	mg
	B2			0.31	mg
	Niacin			2.9	mg
	B6				
	B12				mcg
	C			2	mg
	D				I.U
	E				I.U
	Folic acid				mcg
	K				mcg
Electrolytes					
	Sodium			3	mg
	Potassium			259	mg

NECTARINE   **CAL: 65**

Type: Fruit

Size: medium at approximately 3 per lb.

Description: Very similar in appearance and taste to a peach with the difference being that they have a smooth skin. Nectarines do not do as well as cooked fruits.Peaches are found canned and in pies more often than nectarines. .

NUTRIENTS:

Carbohydrates				16	gms
Proteins				1	gms
Fats				0.1	mg
	Cholesterol			0	mg
	Saturated			0.1	
Water				86	%
Fiber				.54	gms
Minerals					
	Calcium			7	mg
	Iron			0.2	mg
	Magnesium			11	mg
Vitamins					
	A			1000	I.U
	B1			0.02	mg
	B2			0.06	mg
	Niacin			13	mg
	B6			.034	
	B12				mcg
	C			7	mg
	D				I.U
	E				I.U
	Folic acid			5.1	mcg
	K				mcg
Electrolytes					
	Sodium			tr	mg
	Potassium			288	mg

CAL: 25   **OKRA**

Type: Vegetable

Size: Eight, 3 by 5/8" inch pods

Description: These pods are used alone as a vegetable but also in soups and in the Louisiana dish called gumbo. They impart a ropy like consistency to the soups and gumbo. They have traditionally been grown in southern United States and the West Indies. When raw, a half cup has minimum Vitamin K value.

NUTRIENTS:

Carbohydrates				6	gms
Proteins				2	gms
Fats				tr	mg
	Cholesterol			0	mg
	Saturated			tr	
Water				90	%
Fiber					gms
Minerals					
	Calcium			54	mg
	Iron			0.4	mg
	Magnesium				mg
Vitamins					
	A			490	I.U
	B1			0.11	mg
	B2			0.05	mg
	Niacin			0.7	mg
	B6				
	B12				mcg
	C			14	mg
	D				I.U
	E				I.U
	Folic acid				mcg
	K			.32	mcg
Electrolytes					
	Sodium			4	mg
	Potassium			274	mg

Type: Vegetable

Size: 1 small, ripe, canned

Description: Although vegetables are not usually thought of as high in fat, these may be the exception. The ripe ones are matured on the tree and may reach as high as 25 percent fat. The olive has traditionally been thought of as a California product in the United States but are grown in many parts of the world. . Some ripe olives are darker, approaching a black color. Both the green and ripe olives are used alone or in salads, sandwiches etc.

NUTRIENTS:

Carbohydrates				0.20	gms
Proteins				.03	gms
Fats				.34	mg
	Cholesterol			0	mg
	Saturated			.045	
Water				80	%
Fiber					gms
Minerals					
	Calcium			3	mg
	Iron			0.11	mg
	Magnesium				mg
Vitamins					
	A			13	I.U
	B1				mg
	B2				mg
	Niacin				mg
	B6				
	B12				mcg
	C				mg
	D				I.U
	E				I.U
	Folic acid				mcg
	K				mcg
Electrolytes					
	Sodium			28	mg
	Potassium			0	mg

CAL: 55   **ONIIONS**

Type: Vegetable

Size: 1 cup raw,, chopped

Description: Onions are edible bulbs that belong to the Lily family. The many varieties vary in color, shape and size. Most are round and the more popular of these are white, red, or yellow in color. The yellow or "brown" onion tends to have the stronger taste and is frequently used more in cooking while the white and red are used more often in the raw state. Stories abound of the use of onions by the Druids in Egypt and by the Romans in ancient times.

NUTRIENTS:

Carbohydrates				12	gms
Proteins				2	gms
Fats				tr	mg
	Cholesterol			0	mg
	Saturated			0.1	
Water				91	%
Fiber				.94	gms
Minerals					
	Calcium			40	mg
	Iron			0.6	mg
	Magnesium			16	mg
Vitamins					
	A			0	I.U
	B1			0.10	mg
	B2			0.02	mg
	Niacin			0.2	mg
	B6			.18	
	B12				mcg
	C			13	mg
	D				I.U
	E				I.U
	Folic acid			30	mcg
	K				mcg
Electrolytes					
	Sodium			3	mg
	Potassium			248	mg

ORANGE   **CAL: 60**

Type: Fruit

Size: 1 medium at approximately 2-5/8" in diameter.

Description: Possibly the most widely eaten of the citrus fruits. They come in many varieties. The navel Orange is one of the more popular and is known for being virtually seedless. The Valencia is known best for its juice characteristics. It is thought that the fruit was introduced into Europe by way of Asia from India and into California in the early 1870's from Brazil.

NUTRIENTS:

Carbohydrates				15	gms
Proteins				1	gms
Fats				tr	mg
	Cholesterol			0	mg
	Saturated			tr	
Water				87	%
Fiber				0.56	gms
Minerals					
	Calcium			52	mg
	Iron			0.1	mg
	Magnesium			13	mg
Vitamins					
	A			270	I.U
	B1			0.11	mg
	B2			0.05	mg
	Niacin			0.04	mg
	B6			0.079	
	B12				mcg
	C			70	mg
	D				I.U
	E				I.U
	Folic acid			39.7	mcg
	K				mcg
Electrolytes					
	Sodium			tr	mg
	Potassium			237	mg

CAL: 65   **PAPAYA**

Type: Fruit

Size: 1 cup raw of ½ inch cubes

Description: These grow on a rapidly growing tree that resembles a palm. They are somewhat like bananas in that the fruit likes to cluster. The sizes vary from small to up to twenty pounds. Some think that the optimum weight is around three or four pounds. The skin is smooth and the flesh is similar to that of the cantaloupe. There are many seeds in the center. The flesh is generally eaten raw, sometimes with salt and or sugar and some times the seeds are eaten. The seeds are thought to contain papain and felt to be useful as a protein digestive aid.

NUTRIENTS:

Carbohydrates				17	gms
Proteins				1	gms
Fats				tr	mg
	Cholesterol			0	mg
	Saturated			0.1	
Water				86	%
Fiber				1	gms
Minerals					
	Calcium			35	mg
	Iron			0.3	mg
	Magnesium			14	mg
Vitamins					
	A			400	I.U
	B1			0.04	mg
	B2			0.04	mg
	Niacin			0.5	mg
	B6			0.3	
	B12				mcg
	C			92	mg
	D				I.U
	E				I.U
	Folic acid				mcg
	K				mcg
Electrolytes					
	Sodium			9	mg
	Potassium			247	mg

PARSLEY   CAL: 5

Type: Vegetable

Size: 10 sprigs, raw

Description: These sprigs are used as herbs for decorating and adding flavor to dishes. They grow in both the curly and straight form. The curly form is the one with which most people are familiar. The straight leaf form is also known as the chervil. These is an "old wives tale" that the chervil combined in vinegar will stop hiccups.

NUTRIENTS:

Carbohydrates				1	gms
Proteins				tr	gms
Fats				tr	mg
	Cholesterol			0	mg
	Saturated			tr	
Water				88	%
Fiber					gms
Minerals					
	Calcium			13	mg
	Iron			0.6	mg
	Magnesium				mg
Vitamins					
	A			520	I.U
	B1			0.01	mg
	B2			0.01	mg
	Niacin			0.1	mg
	B6				
	B12				mcg
	C			9	mg
	D				I.U
	E				I.U
	Folic acid				mcg
	K			984	mcg
Electrolytes					
	Sodium			4	mg
	Potassium			54	mg

Type: Vegetable

Size: 1 cup

Description: This is a less popular member of root vegetables that belongs to the carrot family. The stronger flavor may account for its lack of favor. They remain fresher if not harvested until wanted as they retain the flavor best. They can however, be frozen without apparent detriment to the flavor. They are generally considered easy to digest.

NUTRIENTS:

Carbohydrates				30	gms
Proteins				2	gms
Fats				tr	mg
	Cholesterol			0	mg
	Saturated			1	
Water				78	%
Fiber					gms
Minerals					
	Calcium			58	mg
	Iron			0.9	mg
	Magnesium				mg
Vitamins					
	A			0	I.U
	B1			0.13	mg
	B2			0.08	mg
	Niacin			1.1	mg
	B6				
	B12				mcg
	C			20	mg
	D				I.U
	E				I.U
	Folic acid				mcg
	K				mcg
Electrolytes					
	Sodium			16	mg
	Potassium			573	mg

Type: Fruit

Size: 1 purple, raw

Description: This fruit, which is also known as the *Maypop*, is the fruit of one of the types of Passion Flowers. The Passion Flower that bears this edible fruit is a vine plant known best in the Southern American States. The fruit is the size of an egg with a tough, purplish skin and a seedy orange colored pulp.

NUTRIENTS:

Carbohydrates				4.21	gms
Proteins				.40	gms
Fats				.13	mg
	Cholesterol			0	mg
	Saturated				
Water				72	%
Fiber				1.97	gms
Minerals					
	Calcium			2	mg
	Iron			0.29	mg
	Magnesium			5	mg
Vitamins					
	A			126	I.U
	B1				mg
	B2			0.02	mg
	Niacin			.27	mg
	B6				
	B12				mcg
	C			5.40	mg
	D				I.U
	E				I.U
	Folic acid				mcg
	K				mcg
Electrolytes					
	Sodium			5	mg
	Potassium			63	mg

Type: Fruit

Size: 1 medium 2 ½ inch in diameter

Description: One of the more popular fruits for both eating fresh or cooked. An ideal ingredient in pies. At one time there were three hundred varieties grown in North America. The current count is unknown. They are generally classified as white or yellow fleshed, or freestone or cling. Similar to appearance to the Nectarine, the skin has a slightly fuzzy texture in contrast to the smooth skin of the Nectarine. Some say that one can find descriptions that resemble Peaches in early Chinese writings.

NUTRIENTS:

Carbohydrates				10	gms
Proteins				1	gms
Fats				tr	mg
	Cholesterol			0	mg
	Saturated			tr	
Water				88	%
Fiber				.6	gms
Minerals					
	Calcium			4	mg
	Iron			0.1	mg
	Magnesium			6	mg
Vitamins					
	A			470	I.U
	B1			0.01	mg
	B2			0.04	mg
	Niacin			0.9	mg
	B6			0.02	
	B12				mcg
	C			6	mg
	D				I.U
	E				I.U
	Folic acid			3.0	mcg
	K				mcg
Electrolytes					
	Sodium			tr	mg
	Potassium			171	mg

PEANUTS   **CAL: 165**

Type: Seed

Size: 1 oz, roasted in oil, salted

Description: The flavor of this kidney shaped nut resembles that of an almond. These nuts are found encased in a hard shell.

NUTRIENTS:

Carbohydrates				5	gms
Proteins				8	gms
Fats				14	mg
	Cholesterol			01.9	mg
	Saturated				
Water				2	%
Fiber				1.49	gms
Minerals					
	Calcium			24	mg
	Iron			0.5	mg
	Magnesium			52	mg
Vitamins					
	A				I.U
	B1			0.8	mg
	B2			0.03	mg
	Niacin			4.2	mg
	B6			.071	
	B12				mcg
	C				mg
	D				I.U
	E				I.U
	Folic acid			35.2	mcg
	K				mcg
Electrolytes					
	Sodium			122	mg
	Potassium			199	mg

Type: Fruit

Size: 1 Bartlett, 2 ½ inch in diameter

Description: The Bartlett pear is one of the most popular of the many pear varieties. The skin is generally yellow with a blush of red and the flesh is white, sweet and quite juicy. The flesh in the middle tends to be grainy in texture. Among the many types, it often last better.

NUTRIENTS:

Carbohydrates				25	gms
Proteins				1	gms
Fats				1	mg
	Cholesterol			0	mg
	Saturated			tr	
Water				84	%
Fiber				2.3	gms
Minerals					
	Calcium			18	mg
	Iron			0.4	mg
	Magnesium				mg
Vitamins					
	A			30	I.U
	B1			0.03	mg
	B2			0.07	mg
	Niacin			0.2	mg
	B6			.03	
	B12				mcg
	C			7	mg
	D				I.U
	E				I.U
	Folic acid			12.1	mcg
	K				mcg
Electrolytes					
	Sodium			Tr	mg
	Potassium			208	mg

PEAS, GREEN   CAL: 115

Type: Legume

Size: 1 cup cooked and drained

Description: These are very popular members of the legumes. They are thought to taste best when cooked soon after picking, in as little water as possible and for as short a time as possible. Both canning and freezing are acceptable methods of preservation if completed immediately after harvesting. Historically speaking there are reports that during the Bronze period there were peas in the Swiss Lake dwellings.

NUTRIENTS:

Carbohydrates				21	gms
Proteins				8	gms
Fats				1	mg
	Cholesterol			0	mg
	Saturated			0.1	
Water				82	%
Fiber				3.7	gms
Minerals					
	Calcium			.34	mg
	Iron			1.6	mg
	Magnesium			63	mg
Vitamins					
	A			1,310	I.U
	B1			0.21	mg
	B2			0.13	mg
	Niacin			1.2	mg
	B6			.35	
	B12				mcg
	C			16	mg
	D				I.U
	E				I.U
	Folic acid			101.3	mcg
	K				mcg
Electrolytes					
	Sodium			372	mg
	Potassium			294	mg

CAL: 190   **PECANS**

Type: Nuts

Size: 1 oz. halves

Description: This popular nut is brown, smooth shelled and olive-shaped. Georgia and Texas are some of the most common growing locations in the United States. Pecan trees have a longevity which can approach 100 years. Consumers find the shelled variety readily available in the markets as it appears to be easier to crack and remove the meat whole when this process is done by commercial means rather than manually.

NUTRIENTS:

Carbohydrates				5	gms
Proteins				2	gms
Fats				19	mg
	Cholesterol			0	mg
	Saturated			1.5	
Water				5	%
Fiber					gms
Minerals					
	Calcium			10	mg
	Iron			0.6	mg
	Magnesium				mg
Vitamins					
	A			40	I.U
	B1			0.24	mg
	B2			0.04	mg
	Niacin			0.3	mg
	B6				
	B12				mcg
	C			1	mg
	D				I.U
	E				I.U
	Folic acid				mcg
	K				mcg
Electrolytes					
	Sodium			tr	mg
	Potassium			111	mg

PEPPERS, SWEET   **CAL: 20**

Type: Vegetable

Size: 1 raw pepper, 1/5th of a pound

Description: These are considered seed pods of the capsicum family. The capsicum family has been used in folk medicine as a topical pain reliever. They are usually found in either the red, yellow or green color. Nutritionally there is little difference. They are generally considered a good source of vitamin C

NUTRIENTS:

Carbohydrates				4	gms
Proteins				1	gms
Fats				tr	mg
	Cholesterol			0	mg
	Saturated			tr	
Water				93	%
Fiber				.32	gms
Minerals					
	Calcium			4	mg
	Iron			0.9	mg
	Magnesium			7	mg
Vitamins					
	A			390	I.U
	B1			0.06	mg
	B2			0.04	mg
	Niacin			0.4	mg
	B6			.184	
	B12				mcg
	C			95	mg
	D				I.U
	E				I.U
	Folic acid			16	mcg
	K				mcg
Electrolytes					
	Sodium			2	mg
	Potassium			144	mg

PERSIMMONS

Type: Fruit

Size: 1 fruit, raw (Japanese)

Description: This fruit comes in two main varieties; American and Japanese. Originally a wild tree in the Southern United States, the fruit is cultivated now for consumption. The American persimmon is generally round in shape with a slightly flattened end while the Japanese variety looks more like a tomato. While immature, the flesh has a very astringent taste but "mellows" and becomes sweet after ripening. Persimmons are more commonly eaten fresh but also lend themselves to drying and freezing.

NUTRIENTS:

Carbohydrates				31.23	gms
Proteins				0.98	gms
Fats				.31	mg
	Cholesterol				mg
	Saturated				
Water				82	%
Fiber				2.49	gms
Minerals					
	Calcium			13	mg
	Iron			0.26	mg
	Magnesium			15	mg
Vitamins					
	A			3,640	I.U
	B1			0.050	mg
	B2			0.034	mg
	Niacin			0.168	mg
	B6				
	B12				mcg
	C			12.6	mg
	D				I.U
	E				I.U
	Folic acid			12.6	mcg
	K				mcg
Electrolytes					
	Sodium			3	mg
	Potassium			270	mg

PINEAPPLE   CAL: 75

Type: Fruit

Size: 1 cup diced, raw

Description: This is most commonly thought of as a Hawaiian fruit. It was probably given its name because of its resemblance to a pine cone. When ripe its surface is a brownish-yellow color and when the leaves are pulled out, it gives a noticeable sweet aroma. Because of a proteolytic enzyme that it contains, fresh pineapple does not mix well with protein products like gelatin. The story goes that the early New England settlers painted the picture of a pineapple over the door as a sign of hospitality.

NUTRIENTS:

Carbohydrates				19	gms
Proteins				1	gms
Fats				1	mg
	Cholesterol			0	mg
	Saturated			tr	
Water				87	%
Fiber				.84	gms
Minerals					
	Calcium			11	mg
	Iron			0.6	mg
	Magnesium			2.1	mg
Vitamins					
	A			40	I.U
	B1			0.14	mg
	B2			0.06	mg
	Niacin			0.7	mg
	B6			0.14	
	B12				mcg
	C			24	mg
	D				I.U
	E				I.U
	Folic acid			1.6	mcg
	K				mcg
Electrolytes					
	Sodium			2	mg
	Potassium			175	mg

Type: Seed

Size: 1 oz. shelled

Description: These are also known as pinion and are one of a variety of edible pine tree nuts. The shells are thin and either brownish yellow or red in color. They are frequently prepared roasted and salted and used in many types of dishes.

NUTRIENTS:

Carbohydrates				5	gms
Proteins				3	gms
Fats				17	mg
	Cholesterol				mg
	Saturated			2.7	
Water				6	%
Fiber					gms
Minerals					
	Calcium			2	mg
	Iron			0.9	mg
	Magnesium				mg
Vitamins					
	A			10	I.U
	B1			0.35	mg
	B2			0.06	mg
	Niacin			1.2	mg
	B6				
	B12				mcg
	C			1	mg
	D				I.U
	E				I.U
	Folic acid				mcg
	K				mcg
Electrolytes					
	Sodium			20	mg
	Potassium			178	mg

PISTACHIO NUTS   **CAL: 165**

Type: Seed

Size: 1 oz. dry, hulled

Description: Though classified as a seed by some, these are often described as green almonds. They come from the reddish pistachio tree. The kernel is oval shaped and the shell becomes brittle and silvery white after it is salted . The most popular way of consuming them are when either eaten raw or after roasting and salting. At one time it is said, that they were a courtesy offering to visitors in the Far East.

NUTRIENTS:

Carbohydrates				7	gms
Proteins				6	gms
Fats				14	mg
	Cholesterol			0	mg
	Saturated			1.7	
Water				4	%
Fiber					gms
Minerals					
	Calcium			38	mg
	Iron			1.9	mg
	Magnesium				mg
Vitamins					
	A			70	I.U
	B1			0.23	mg
	B2			0.05	mg
	Niacin			0.3	mg
	B6				
	B12				mcg
	C			tr	mg
	D				I.U
	E				I.U
	Folic acid				mcg
	K				mcg
Electrolytes					
	Sodium			2	mg
	Potassium			310	mg

Type: Fruit

Size: 1 cup cooked

Description: This is one of several types of bananas. It is not eaten raw and when baked or roasted has the texture of a potato. Sometimes it is dried and ground and used as a meal in baking cakes and breads. It has been seen commonly in some of the Caribbean Island dishes.

NUTRIENTS:

Carbohydrates				57	gms
Proteins				1	gms
Fats				tr	mg
	Cholesterol			0	mg
	Saturated			0.1	
Water				67	%
Fiber					gms
Minerals					
	Calcium			5	mg
	Iron			1.1	mg
	Magnesium			49	mg
Vitamins					
	A			2,020	I.U
	B1			0.09	mg
	B2			0.10	mg
	Niacin			1.2	mg
	B6			.37	
	B12				mcg
	C			33	mg
	D				I.U
	E				I.U
	Folic acid			40	mcg
	K				mcg
Electrolytes					
	Sodium			7	mg
	Potassium			893	mg

PLUM   **CAL: 35**

Type: Fruit

Size: 1 raw

Description: There are several varieties of plums today. They may be eaten raw or cooked, and plum jam is a favorite among many home cooks. In Southern California they are often an early summer fruit with a short harvesting period. Modern methods of farming and present day transportation however, now make it available almost year round in supermarkets.

NUTRIENTS:

Carbohydrates				9	gms
Proteins				1	gms
Fats				tr	mg
	Cholesterol			0	mg
	Saturated			tr	
Water				85	%
Fiber				.4	gms
Minerals					
	Calcium			3	mg
	Iron			0.1	mg
	Magnesium			4	mg
Vitamins					
	A			210	I.U
	B1			0.03	mg
	B2			0.06	mg
	Niacin			0.3	mg
	B6			.05	
	B12				mcg
	C			6	mg
	D				I.U
	E				I.U
	Folic acid				mcg
	K				mcg
Electrolytes					
	Sodium			tr	mg
	Potassium			114	mg

CAL: 104

Type: Fruit

Size: 1 raw

Description: This fruit is messy to eat out of hand as it encloses many seeds. The edible flesh is reddish pink in color and quite juicy. The taste is sweet with an acid touch. The juice has traditionally been captured and sold as grenadine syrup but today can now be found in many markets as a beverage labeled simply Pomegranate juice. . The pomegranate is about the size of an orange but ranges in color from yellow to purplish. The rind is thick and leathery.

NUTRIENTS:

Carbohydrates				26.4	gms
Proteins				1.47	gms
Fats				.46	mg
	Cholesterol				mg
	Saturated				
Water				81	%
Fiber				.31	gms
Minerals					
	Calcium			5	mg
	Iron			0.5	mg
	Magnesium				mg
Vitamins					
	A				I.U
	B1			0.05	mg
	B2			0.05	mg
	Niacin			0.05	mg
	B6			16	
	B12				mcg
	C			9.4	mg
	D				I.U
	E				I.U
	Folic acid				mcg
	K				mcg
Electrolytes					
	Sodium			5	mg
	Potassium			399	mg

POTATO, SWEET   CAL: 115

Type: Vegetable

Size: 1 baked potato, with peel, approximately ½ lb.

Description: Another of the tuber types of vegetables. Unlike the white potato the shape tends to be tapered at both ends, the flesh yellowish orange in color and when cooked is sweeter to taste.

NUTRIENTS:

Carbohydrates				28	gms
Proteins				2	gms
Fats				tr	mg
	Cholesterol			0	mg
	Saturated			tr	
Water				73	%
Fiber					gms
Minerals					
	Calcium			32	mg
	Iron			0.5	mg
	Magnesium				mg
Vitamins					
	A			24,880	I.U
	B1			0.08	mg
	B2			0.14	mg
	Niacin				mg
	B6				
	B12				mcg
	C			28	mg
	D				I.U
	E				I.U
	Folic acid				mcg
	K				mcg
Electrolytes					
	Sodium			11	mg
	Potassium			397	mg

CAL: 145   **POTATO, WHITE**

Type: Vegetable

Size: 1 baked potato, flesh only, 1/4th

Description: This vegetable is a staple in the diet in many countries, particularly in the United States. This edible tuber is prepared in many ways including boiling, baking and frying. There are several verities of white potatoes depending on size, color, texture when cooked and the texture of the skin. There is not a notable nutritional difference but they do not fare equally well in all methods of preparation. The calorie count is increased in relation to the items added in preparation.

NUTRIENTS:

Carbohydrates				34	gms
Proteins				3	gms
Fats				tr	mg
	Cholesterol			0	mg
	Saturated			tr	
Water				75	%
Fiber					gms
Minerals					
	Calcium			8	mg
	Iron			0.5	mg
	Magnesium				mg
Vitamins					
	A			0	I.U
	B1			0.16	mg
	B2			0.03	mg
	Niacin			2.2	mg
	B6				
	B12				mcg
	C			20	mg
	D				I.U
	E				I.U
	Folic acid				mcg
	K				mcg
Electrolytes					
	Sodium			8	mg
	Potassium			610	mg

Type: Fruit

Size: 1 raw

Description: This is classified as a fruit but belongs to the cactus family. The prickly pear type is the best known of the many cacti and is edible. The fruit are shaped like pears or figs and are called by some the Nopal or Indian Fig. The fruit grows on the edge of the leaf like joints which are flat. The plant is also used as feed for livestock. In Mexico and Central America, one edible variety is known as *tuna*.

NUTRIENTS:

Carbohydrates				0.86	gms
Proteins				75	gms
Fats				.53	mg
	Cholesterol				mg
	Saturated				
Water				87	%
Fiber				1.87	gms
Minerals					
	Calcium			58	mg
	Iron			.31	mg
	Magnesium			88	mg
Vitamins					
	A			53	I.U
	B1			0.01	mg
	B2			0.06	mg
	Niacin			0.47	mg
	B6				
	B12				mcg
	C			14	mg
	D				I.U
	E				I.U
	Folic acid				mcg
	K				mcg
Electrolytes					
	Sodium			6	mg
	Potassium			226	mg

CAL: 115   **PRUNES**

Type: Fruit

Size: 5 large, uncooked

Description: These are actually dried plums which are left on the tree to ripen and fall of their own accord. After harvesting some are pitted but many are sold with the seeds intact. Many people find them useful as a "natural" laxative source.

NUTRIENTS:

Carbohydrates				31	gms
Proteins				1	gms
Fats				tr	mg
	Cholesterol			0	mg
	Saturated			tr	
Water				32	%
Fiber				.95	gms
Minerals					
	Calcium			25	mg
	Iron			1.2	mg
	Magnesium			21	mg
Vitamins					
	A			970	I.U
	B1			0.04	mg
	B2			0.08	mg
	Niacin			1.0	mg
	B6			.25	
	B12				mcg
	C			2	mg
	D				I.U
	E				I.U
	Folic acid			.65	mcg
	K				mcg
Electrolytes					
	Sodium			2	mg
	Potassium			365	mg

PUMPKIN   **CAL: 50**

Type: Vegetable

Size: 1 cup cooked, from raw and mashed

Description: Like the squash, this vegetable grows on a vine and belongs to the gourd family. These round, orange colored vegetables grow quite large. Pumpkin pie is the presentation most well known for the flesh of this gourd. It is very similar in taste to the sweet potato pie. when prepared in this manner with sugar and spices

NUTRIENTS:

Carbohydrates				12	gms
Proteins				2	gms
Fats				tr	mg
	Cholesterol			0	mg
	Saturated			0.1	
Water				90	%
Fiber					gms
Minerals					
	Calcium			37	mg
	Iron			3.4	mg
	Magnesium				mg
Vitamins					
	A			2,650	I.U
	B1			0.08	mg
	B2			0.19	mg
	Niacin			1.0	mg
	B6				
	B12				mcg
	C			12	mg
	D				I.U
	E				I.U
	Folic acid				mcg
	K			40	mcg
Electrolytes					
	Sodium			2	mg
	Potassium			564	mg

CAL: 5   **RADICCHIO**

Type: Vegetable

Size: ½ cup shredded

Description: This vegetable grows quickly, forming a white root that is tender to taste. It is often boiled or steamed and eaten as a vegetable It is also sliced and consumed in salads. They appear in both red and white colors. The young ones are most tender while the older and larger ones tend to be tough with a strong flavor.

NUTRIENTS:

Carbohydrates				90	gms
Proteins				.29	gms
Fats				.05	mg
	Cholesterol			0	mg
	Saturated				
Water				93	%
Fiber					gms
Minerals					
	Calcium			4	mg
	Iron				mg
	Magnesium			3	mg
Vitamins					
	A			5	I.U
	B1				mg
	B2				mg
	Niacin			0.5	mg
	B6			.011	
	B12				mcg
	C			1.6	mg
	D				I.U
	E				I.U
	Folic acid				mcg
	K				mcg
Electrolytes					
	Sodium			4	mg
	Potassium			60	mg

113

Type: Vegetable

Size: 4 , raw

Description: It is the root of these vegetables that are consumed raw, usually in salads or often as garnishes. They are found in various colors (red and white), sizes and shapes (round, oval and long). They have a tendency to a sharp taste.

NUTRIENTS:

Carbohydrates				1	gms
Proteins				tr	gms
Fats				tr	mg
	Cholesterol			0	mg
	Saturated			tr	
Water				95	%
Fiber				.48	gms
Minerals					
	Calcium			4	mg
	Iron			0,1	mg
	Magnesium			8	mg
Vitamins					
	A			tr	I.U
	B1			tr	mg
	B2			0.01	mg
	Niacin			0.1	mg
	B6			.052	
	B12				mcg
	C			4	mg
	D				I.U
	E				I.U
	Folic acid			8	mcg
	K				mcg
Electrolytes					
	Sodium			4	mg
	Potassium			42	mg

114

Type: Fruit

Size: 1 cup seedless, uncooked

Description: These are dried grapes frequently of the Muscat or Thompson variety. At one time California was the largest producer of raisins.

NUTRIENTS:

Carbohydrates				115	gms
Proteins				5	gms
Fats				1	mg
	Cholesterol			0	mg
	Saturated			0.2	
Water				15	%
Fiber				2	gms
Minerals					
	Calcium			71	mg
	Iron			3.0	mg
	Magnesium			51	mg
Vitamins					
	A			10	I.U
	B1			0.23	mg
	B2			0.13	mg
	Niacin			1.2	mg
	B6			.47	
	B12				mcg
	C			5	mg
	D				I.U
	E				I.U
	Folic acid			4.8	mcg
	K				mcg
Electrolytes					
	Sodium			17	mg
	Potassium			1,089	mg

RASPBERRIES   CAL: 60

Type: Fruit

Size: 1 cup uncooked

Description: Most commonly thought of as early summer fruit, they do not hold up well and are easily bruised or crushed. Today due to modern technology and transportation, they can be found sometimes year around. These berries freeze well and are commonly made into jams. They are found in both red and black varieties.

NUTRIENTS:

Carbohydrates				14	gms
Proteins				1	gms
Fats				1	mg
	Cholesterol				mg
	Saturated			tr	
Water				87	%
Fiber				3.7	gms
Minerals					
	Calcium			27	mg
	Iron			1.6	mg
	Magnesium			22	mg
Vitamins					
	A			160	I.U
	B1			0.04	mg
	B2			0.11	mg
	Niacin			1.1	mg
	B6			.07	
	B12				mcg
	C			31	mg
	D				I.U
	E				I.U
	Folic acid				mcg
	K				mcg
Electrolytes					
	Sodium			tr	mg
	Potassium			187	mg

CAL: 280   **RHUBARB**

Type: Fruit

Size: 1 cup of chopped stalks, cooked, with sugar added.

Description: This plant carries several cautions. Both the leaves and the stalk contain oxalic acid. While the stalk is not felt to be harmful in the quantity eaten most often, the leaves are possibly deadly. The taste is quite bitter alone therefore is almost NEVER eaten without adding quite a bit of sugar in the cooking. It is a common ingredient in pies especially when combined with strawberries. For some individuals it has a laxative effect.

NUTRIENTS:

Carbohydrates				75	gms
Proteins				1	gms
Fats				tr	mg
	Cholesterol			0	mg
	Saturated			tr	
Water				68	%
Fiber				1.92	gms
Minerals					
	Calcium			348	mg
	Iron			0.5	mg
	Magnesium			30	mg
Vitamins					
	A			170	I.U
	B1			0.04	mg
	B2			0.06	mg
	Niacin			0.5	mg
	B6			.5	
	B12				mcg
	C			8	mg
	D				I.U
	E				I.U
	Folic acid			12.7	mcg
	K				mcg
Electrolytes					
	Sodium			2	mg
	Potassium			230	mg

ROSELLE

Type: Fruit

Size: 1 cup raw

Description: The edible parts of this bushy, annual hibiscus plant are the seed pods, flowers and stems. The plant is common in the tropics and the southern United States. The pods look like those of the okra but are red in color and acid to taste. The seeds are used for sauces and jellies while the flowers are used in pies, puddings, jams and jellies. The juice of the stems is used in beverages as well as in jellies. In Florida , Roselle may be found under the name Jamaican Sorrel.

NUTRIENTS:

Carbohydrates				6.45	gms
Proteins				55	gms
Fats				36	mg
	Cholesterol				mg
	Saturated				
Water				85	%
Fiber				.65	gms
Minerals					
	Calcium			123	mg
	Iron			0.84	mg
	Magnesium			29	mg
Vitamins					
	A			163	I.U
	B1				mg
	B2			0.01	mg
	Niacin			0.17	mg
	B6				
	B12				mcg
	C			6.8	mg
	D				I.U
	E				I.U
	Folic acid				mcg
	K				mcg
Electrolytes					
	Sodium			3	mg
	Potassium			118	mg

CAL: 140   **SAPODILLA**

Type: Fruit

Size: 1 fruit, raw

Description: The Evergreen species which produces chicle, bears this fruit. This thin skinned, russet colored fruit is similar in shape to an apple. The ripe flesh is soft, yellowish brown in color and granular in texture Spicy and sweet, it is most commonly eaten fresh.

NUTRITENS:

Carbohydrates				33.9	gms
Proteins				.74	gms
Fats				1.87	mg
	Cholesterol				mg
	Saturated				
Water				78	%
Fiber				2.38	gms
Minerals					
	Calcium			36	mg
	Iron			1.36	mg
	Magnesium				mg
Vitamins					
	A			102	I.U
	B1				mg
	B2			0.03	mg
	Niacin			0.34	mg
	B6			.06	
	B12				mcg
	C			25	mg
	D				I.U
	E				I.U
	Folic acid				mcg
	K				mcg
Electrolytes					
	Sodium			20	mg
	Potassium			328	mg

Type: Fruit

Size: 1 fruit, raw

Description: Previously known as a Central American fruit they are also grown in Florida. This fruit is found in two colors; white and green. The white variety is oval in shape and has a thick, woody skin. Its flesh is pulpy in nature and reddish in color. This one has a single seed which is large. The green variety is rare. It is oblong in shape with a thin greenish skin. The interior is cinnamon colored. They are both eaten mainly as fresh fruit.

NUTRIENTS:

Carbohydrates				76	gms
Proteins				4.8	gms
Fats				1.35	mg
	Cholesterol				mg
	Saturated				
Water				62	%
Fiber					gms
				4.28	
Minerals					
	Calcium				88	mg
	Iron				2.25	mg
	Magnesium				68	mg
Vitamins					
	A				923	I.U
	B1				0.02	mg
	B2				0.04	mg
	Niacin				4.05	mg
	B6					
	B12					mcg
	C				45	mg
	D					I.U
	E					I.U
	Folic acid					mcg
	K					mcg
Electrolytes					
	Sodium				21	mg
	Potassium				773	mg

CAL: 45   **SAUERKRAUT**

Type: Vegetable

Size: 1 cup canned

Description: Shredded cabbage that has been fermented. It is usually made from the white cabbage and has a light beige color and a crisp texture. Traditionally thought of as a Russian or German dish.

NUTRIENTS:

Carbohydrates				10	gms
Proteins				2	gms
Fats				tr	mg
	Cholesterol			0	mg
	Saturated			0.1	
Water				93	%
Fiber					gms
Minerals					
	Calcium			71	mg
	Iron			3.5	mg
	Magnesium				mg
Vitamins					
	A			40	I.U
	B1			0.05	mg
	B2			0.05	mg
	Niacin			0.3	mg
	B6				
	B12				mcg
	C			35	mg
	D				I.U
	E				I.U
	Folic acid				mcg
	K				mcg
Electrolytes					
	Sodium			1,560	mg
	Potassium			564	mg

Type: Seed

Size: 1 tbsp dry, hulled

Description: This annual plant is an oblong four celled seed capsule and it contains many small flat seeds. The seeds vary in color from white to brown and are utilized many ways in cooking. One of the most popular uses of this plant is to extract the seed oil and use it in cooking. Sesame oil is a common ingredient in Oriental style dishes. This seed also carries the name *benne* in some places. One story states that sesame seeds were introduced into the United States via Florida by African Americans.

NUTRIENTS:

Carbohydrates				1	gms
Proteins				2	gms
Fats				4	mg
	Cholesterol			0	mg
	Saturated			0.6	
Water				5	%
Fiber					gms
Minerals					
	Calcium			11	mg
	Iron			5.1	mg
	Magnesium				mg
Vitamins					
	A			10	I.U
	B1			0.06	mg
	B2			0.01	mg
	Niacin			0.4	mg
	B6				
	B12				mcg
	C				mg
	D				I.U
	E				I.U
	Folic acid				mcg
	K				mcg
Electrolytes					
	Sodium			3	mg
	Potassium			33	mg

Type: Fruit

Size: 1 cup of pulp

Description: This is the fruit of an evergreen tree of the custard-apple family. It is found in Florida and other sub-tropical regions. The fruit is large with each weighing over a pound. The skin is dark green in color, thick in texture and with many fleshy spines. It is shaped somewhat like a pineapple. The pulp is white and acidic to taste. When pureed and sweetened, it is a favorite in frozen desserts.

NUTRIENTS:

Carbohydrates				38	gms
Proteins				2.25	gms
Fats				.68	mg
	Cholesterol				mg
	Saturated				
Water				81	%
Fiber				2.5	gms
Minerals					
	Calcium			32	mg
	Iron			1.35	mg
	Magnesium			46	mg
Vitamins					
	A			5	I.U
	B1			0.16	mg
	B2			0.11	mg
	Niacin			2.02	mg
	B6			.13	
	B12				mcg
	C			46	mg
	D				I.U
	E				I.U
	Folic acid				mcg
	K				mcg
Electrolytes					
	Sodium			31	mg
	Potassium			626	mg

SPINACH   **CAL: 40**

Type: Vegetable

Size: 1 cup cooked and drained

Description: This leafy vegetable is possibly the most popular of the "greens" type vegetables. Often touted as being very high in iron it became famous as the food that made "Popeye" the sailor man strong. Through it is still considered a nutritious product, it's claims to fame are probably overrated. Some of its nutrients i.e. Calcium and iron are not totally absorbable. It is served both raw, as a salad vegetable and cooked.

NUTRIENTS:

Carbohydrates				7	gms
Proteins				5	gms
Fats				tr	mg
	Cholesterol			0	mg
	Saturated			tr	
Water				91	%
Fiber					gms
Minerals					
	Calcium			245	mg
	Iron			6.4	mg
	Magnesium				mg
Vitamins					
	A			14,740	I.U
	B1			0.17	mg
	B2			0.42	mg
	Niacin			0.9	mg
	B6				
	B12				mcg
	C			18	mg
	D				I.U
	E				I.U
	Folic acid				mcg
	K			888	mcg
Electrolytes					
	Sodium			126	mg
	Potassium			839	mg

SQUASH, SUMMER   **CAL: 35**

Type: Vegetable

Size: 1 cup cooked, and drained

Description: This group of squash include names such zucchini and patty pan. They are characterized by a crookneck, rough pod and cream colored flesh. The entire plant is eaten including the rind, seeds and flesh. They are often steamed or boiled. Another method of preparation often called tempura, is seen when the vegetable is dipped in egg and crumbs or flour mixtures and deep fried.

NUTRIENTS:

Carbohydrates				8	gms
Proteins				2	gms
Fats				1	mg
	Cholesterol			0	mg
	Saturated			0.1	
Water				94	%
Fiber					gms
Minerals					
	Calcium			49	mg
	Iron			0.6	mg
	Magnesium				mg
Vitamins					
	A			520	I.U
	B1			0.08	mg
	B2			0.07	mg
	Niacin			0.9	mg
	B6				
	B12				mcg
	C			10	mg
	D				I.U
	E				I.U
	Folic acid				mcg
	K				mcg
Electrolytes					
	Sodium			2	mg
	Potassium			346	mg

Type: Vegetable

Size: 1 cup baked

Description: The winter squash tend to be larger than the summer type and they are not as perishable. The peels or rinds are less multicolored and the seeds are usually discarded. To find these in the market look for names such as *Hubbard, Delicious and Germaine Mammoth*.

NUTRIENTS:

Carbohydrates				18	gms
Proteins				2	gms
Fats				1	mg
	Cholesterol			0	mg
	Saturated			0.3	
Water				89	%
Fiber				0.7	gms
Minerals					
	Calcium			29	mg
	Iron			0.7	mg
	Magnesium				mg
Vitamins					
	A			7,290	I.U
	B1			0.17	mg
	B2			0.05	mg
	Niacin			1.4	mg
	B6				
	B12				mcg
	C			20	mg
	D				I.U
	E				I.U
	Folic acid				mcg
	K				mcg
Electrolytes					
	Sodium			2	mg
	Potassium			896	mg

Type: Fruit

Size: 1 cup whole, fresh

Description: This red, sweet berry, is found growing in both the wild and cultivated state. The growing season is short but modern technology appears to have extended it somewhat. It is excellent as both a fresh food or when cooked in pies, or made into jams and jellies. They freeze well.

NUTRIENTS:

Carbohydrates				10	gms
Proteins				1	gms
Fats				tr	mg
	Cholesterol			0	mg
	Saturated			tr	
Water				92	%
Fiber				.63	gms
Minerals					
	Calcium			21	mg
	Iron			0.6	mg
	Magnesium			16	mg
Vitamins					
	A			40	I.U
	B1			0.03	mg
	B2			0.10	mg
	Niacin			0.3	mg
	B6			.08	
	B12				mcg
	C			84	mg
	D				I.U
	E				I.U
	Folic acid			26.4	mcg
	K				mcg
Electrolytes					
	Sodium			1	mg
	Potassium			247	mg

Type: Seed

Size: 1 oz, dried and hulled

Description: These seeds are harvested from the flower that bears the name. The flower is normally large and is a popular item for florist and farmers alike. Some varieties are perennials but others are planed anew each year from seed. The flower is easily recognized as it has bright yellow petals surrounding a dark brown center.

NUTRIENTS:

Carbohydrates				5	gms
Proteins				6	gms
Fats				14	mg
	Cholesterol			0	mg
	Saturated			1.5	
Water				5	%
Fiber					gms
Minerals					
	Calcium			33	mg
	Iron			1.9	mg
	Magnesium				mg
Vitamins					
	A			10	I.U
	B1			0.65	mg
	B2			0.07	mg
	Niacin			1.3	mg
	B6				
	B12				mcg
	C			tr	mg
	D				I.U
	E				I.U
	Folic acid				mcg
	K				mcg
Electrolytes					
	Sodium			1	mg
	Potassium			195	mg

Type: Fruit

Size: 1 cup pulp

Description: It is the product of the pulp of this plump, brown pod that is consumed as flavoring for preserves, beverages, chutneys, curries and sauces. The tree originally seen in East Africa is now common in the United States; particularly Florida. The edible portion is the pulp which is found inside the brittle shell of the pod. The pulp is sweet though somewhat acidic in flavor. In the pulp are embedded the flat, glossy seeds. One method of preparation is to seal the seeds and pulp in hot syrup.

NUTRIENTS:

Carbohydrates				75	gms
Proteins				3.3	gms
Fats				72	mg
	Cholesterol			0	mg
	Saturated			.33	
Water				31	%
Fiber				6.12	gms
Minerals					
	Calcium			1	mg
	Iron			3.4	mg
	Magnesium			110	mg
Vitamins					
	A			36	I.U
	B1			.51	mg
	B2			.18	mg
	Niacin			2.33	mg
	B6			.08	
	B12				mcg
	C			4.2	mg
	D				I.U
	E				I.U
	Folic acid				mcg
	K				mcg
Electrolytes					
	Sodium			33	mg
	Potassium			753	mg

Type: Fruit

Size: 1 2-3/8⁴ inch diameter, fresh

Description: These orange colored citrus fruits are characterized by the ease with which they are peeled in contrast to the usual orange. They are thought to have originated in China and this led to their being called Mandarins by some. Today the mandarin is frequently a smaller variety and is often canned.

NUTRIENTS:

Carbohydrates				9	gms
Proteins				1	gms
Fats				tr	mg
	Cholesterol			0	mg
	Saturated			tr	
Water				88	%
Fiber				.28	gms
Minerals					
	Calcium			12	mg
	Iron			0.1	mg
	Magnesium			10	mg
Vitamins					
	A			770	I.U
	B1			0.09	mg
	B2			0.02	mg
	Niacin			0.1	mg
	B6			.06	
	B12				mcg
	C			26	mg
	D				I.U
	E				I.U
	Folic acid				mcg
	K				mcg
Electrolytes					
	Sodium			1	mg
	Potassium			132	mg

Type: Vegetable

Size: 1 fresh, 2-3/5ᵗʰ inch diameter

Description: Listed here as a vegetable, there are those who will argue the point and proclaim these as fruit. The traditional concept of this vegetable is that of a round and beautiful red item. In reality the colors range from green to yellow. The shapes are round to elongated and the sizes from quite small to beefsteak. Freshly picked, vine ripened tomatoes are touted as sweet and delicious. Tomatoes lend themselves to any number of dishes and to being consumed both fresh and cooked. They preserve well as canned products.

NUTRIENTS:

Carbohydrates				5	gms
Proteins				1	gms
Fats				tr	mg
	Cholesterol			0	mg
	Saturated			Tr	
Water				94	%
Fiber				.81	gms
Minerals					
	Calcium			9	mg
	Iron			0.6	mg
	Magnesium			13	mg
Vitamins					
	A			1,390	I.U
	B1			0.07	mg
	B2			0.06	mg
	Niacin			0.7	mg
	B6			.09	
	B12				mcg
	C			22	mg
	D				I.U
	E				I.U
	Folic acid			.18	mcg
	K				mcg
Electrolytes					
	Sodium			10	mg
	Potassium			255	mg

Type: Vegetable

Size: 1 cup cooked, diced

Description: One of the root type vegetables. Both the leaves and the root are edible but neither are outstanding in nutritive value. The roots are seen in both white and yellow color and are eaten raw and cooked.

NUTRIENTS:

Carbohydrates				8	gms
Proteins				1	gms
Fats				tr	mg
	Cholesterol			0	mg
	Saturated			tr	
Water				94	%
Fiber					gms
Minerals					
	Calcium			34	mg
	Iron			0.3	mg
	Magnesium				mg
Vitamins					
	A			0	I.U
	B1			0.04	mg
	B2			0.04	mg
	Niacin			0.5	mg
	B6				
	B12				mcg
	C			18	mg
	D				I.U
	E				I.U
	Folic acid				mcg
	K				mcg
Electrolytes					
	Sodium			78	mg
	Potassium			211	mg

CAL: 170   **WALNUTS**

Type: Seed

Size: 1 oz chopped

Description: These are usually of two colors, the black and the white. Nutritionally, there is not a great amount of difference between them. Both have green hulls. The shell of the black is more difficult to crack than the white. The white are often called English or Persian. In a few instances, walnuts may discolor the product when combined with other foods. The shells have been made into charcoal in the past. It is said that the Romans called walnuts the "nut of the Gods."

NUTRIENTS:

Carbohydrates				3	gms
Proteins				7	gms
Fats				16	mg
	Cholesterol			0	mg
	Saturated			1.0	
Water				4	%
Fiber					gms
Minerals					
	Calcium			27	mg
	Iron			0.7	mg
	Magnesium				mg
Vitamins					
	A			80	I.U
	B1			0.06	mg
	B2			0.03	mg
	Niacin			0.2	mg
	B6				
	B12				mcg
	C			tr	mg
	D				I.U
	E				I.U
	Folic acid				mcg
	K				mcg
Electrolytes					
	Sodium			tr	mg
	Potassium			149	mg

WATER CHESTNUTS   **CAL: 70**

Type: Vegetable

Size: 1 cup canned

Description: These are another type of chestnut but are more commonly thought of as vegetables rather than as nuts. They may actually derive from one of several sources. They can be the bulb of a rush like plant or they can be also the fruit kernels of some types of aquatic plants that float. They are commonly used in Oriental cooking.

NUTRIENTS:

Carbohydrates				17	gms
Proteins				1	gms
Fats				tr	mg
	Cholesterol			0	mg
	Saturated			tr	
Water				86	%
Fiber					gms
Minerals					
	Calcium			6	mg
	Iron			1.2	mg
	Magnesium				mg
Vitamins					
	A			10	I.U
	B1			0.02	mg
	B2			0.03	mg
	Niacin			0.5	mg
	B6				
	B12				mcg
	C			2	mg
	D				I.U
	E				I.U
	Folic acid				mcg
	K				mcg
Electrolytes					
	Sodium			11	mg
	Potassium			165	mg

Type: Fruit

Size: 1 piece ,4 by 8 inch wedge with rind and seeds

Description: This is another of the melon fruits that grows on running vines. It comes in all sizes and is either oval or round shaped. The skin is smooth with a dark green color or with stripes. It usually has many rows of seeds but today a "seedless" variety can be found in some markets. The term is a misnomer because some seeds can almost always be found even in the seedless but the quantity is less.

NUTRIENTS:

Carbohydrates				35	gms
Proteins				3	gms
Fats				2	mg
	Cholesterol			0	mg
	Saturated				
Water				92	%
Fiber				1.45	gms
Minerals					
	Calcium			39	mg
	Iron			0.8	mg
	Magnesium			52	mg
Vitamins					
	A			1,760	I.U
	B1			0.39	mg
	B2			0.10	mg
	Niacin			1.0	mg
	B6			0.7	
	B12				mcg
	C			46	mg
	D				I.U
	E				I.U
	Folic acid			10.4	mcg
	K				mcg
Electrolytes					
	Sodium			10	mg
	Potassium			559	mg

RECOMMENDED DAILY ALLOWANCES
aka RDA

This terminology is rarely used today but is included anyway because it is still a much simpler way to think about the nutritional value of foods. It is also an easier way to utilize the counts expressed in these pages. Today this information is best found under the terms ___DIETARY REFERENCE INTAKES (DRI)___[2]. In this resource from the National Academy of Science the data is quite detailed, voluminous and specific. It would be inappropriate and inefficient to attempt to duplicate its information here. As advised in the Preface, anyone who needs this data for serious nutritional reasons, SHOUD NOT rely on ANY number found in these pages and should seek current, professional, nutritional counseling.

The RDA numbers listed here have changed and are provided only as a guide for thinking about what to eat. These numbers give the reader a ballpark for choice and are not to be construed as specific medical guidance.

Men

Age 19 - 22	21-50	51,
Weight 154	154	154
Height 70 inches	70	70
Daily Calories 2,900	2,700	2,400
Protein 56gms	56gms	56gms

Vitamins and Minerals

Calcium 800 mgs	800 mgs	800 mgs
Iron 10 mgs	10 mgs	10 mgs
Vit A 5,000 I.U	5,000 I.U.	5,000 I.U.
Vit B1 1.5 mgs	1.4 mgs	1.2 mgs
Vit B2 1.7 mgs	1.6 mgs	1.4 mgs
Niacin 19 mgs	18 mgs	16 mgs
Cit C 60 mg	60 mgs	60 mgs

Women

Age 19 –22	23 –50	51+
Proteins 44gms	44 gms	44 gms

Vitamins and Minerals

Calcium 800 mgs	80 mgs	800 mgs
Iron 18 mgs	18 mgs	10 mgs
Vit A 4,000 I.U.	4,000 I.U.	4,000 I.U.
Vit B1 1.1 mgs	1.0 mgs	1.0 mgs
Vit B2 1.3 mgs	1.2 mgs	1.2 mgs
Niacin 14 mgs	13 mgs	13 mgs
Vit C 60 mgs	60 mgs	60 mgs

---

[2] See addendum under Nation Academy of Science

TOP TEN

CALORIES

FOOD	QUANTITY	VALUE
Figs	10 dried	475
Raisins	1 cup	435
Cranberry Sauce (with sugar)	1 cup	420
Chestnuts	1 cup	350
Avocado	12 gms	305
Coconut	12 gms	285
Rhubarb (Cooked with sugar)	1 cup	280
Beans, Pinto	1 cup	265
Beans, Lima	1 cup	260
Soybeans	1 cup	235